CANCER ETIOLOGY, DIAGNOSIS AND TREATMENTS

NON-SMALL CELL LUNG CANCER

NEW RESEARCH

CANCER ETIOLOGY, DIAGNOSIS AND TREATMENTS

Additional books in this series can be found on Nova's website under the Series tab.

Additional E-books in this series can be found on Nova's website under the E-book tab.

CANCER ETIOLOGY, DIAGNOSIS AND TREATMENTS

NON-SMALL CELL LUNG CANCER

NEW RESEARCH

LINA PASQUARIELLO
EDITOR

New York

For permission to use material from this book please contact us:
Telephone 631-231-7269; Fax 631-231-8175
Web Site: http://www.novapublishers.com

Library of Congress Cataloging-in-Publication Data

ISBN: 978-1-62417-804-7

Library of Congress Control Number: 2012955912

Published by Nova Science Publishers, Inc. † New York

Contents

Preface

In this book, the authors present current research in the study of non-small cell lung cancer. Topics discussed include the preclinical and clinical advances of epigenetics in lung cancer; therapeutic antibodies and non-coding RNAs (ncRNAs) in non-small cell lung cancer; molecular profiling in lung cancer specimens leads to targeted therapeutic options in patients with non-small cell lung carcinoma; the role of radiation dose escalation in the treatment of stage III locally advanced inoperable non-small cell lung cancer; and mechanisms of resistance to EGFR inhibitors.

Chapter 1 - Lung cancer is the leading cause of cancer-related deaths in industrialized countries and non small cell lung cancer (NSCLC) accounts for 85% of all lung cancers. Cisplatin doublet based chemotherapy, which is recommended regimen in first line therapy in advanced or metastatic NSCLC, improves survival but in low proportion. Monoclonal antibodies (mAbs) are a novel promising therapy class used with great results in inflammatory diseases such as rheumatoid arthritis. Antibodies are natural proteins with modular structure, specific pharmacodynamics and pharmacokinetics and possibly produced against any antigens, thus giving them several advantages over small drug therapeutics. In solid tumors, therapeutic mAbs improved progression free survival (PFS) and overall survival (OS) of patients with breast and colon cancers and had considerably changed the treatment in clinical practice. In NSCLC, bevacizumab, an anti-VEGF mAb and cetuximab, an anti-EGFR mAb, are the most studied antibodies. Bevacizumab acts on angiognenesis and improved PFS of non squamous NSCLC but in low proportion as shown in two large phase III trials. It was approved by European Medicines Agency (EMEA) and Food and Drug administration (FDA) as a first line therapy in combination with cisplatin doublet chemotherapy. Cetuximab slightly enhanced OS but did not improve PFS in two large phase III trials. These results added to high adverse effect lead to cetuximab refusal by EMEA and FDA in NSCLC. At first glance, the results of mAbs in NSCLC are somewhat disappointing, in contrast to the benefits obtained with mAb treatments in other solid tumors. However, many other mAbs directed against novel targets, such as IGF1-R or CTLA-4, and new mAbs targeting VEGFR and EGFR pathways with different pharmacodymamical and pharmacokinetic properties are under evaluation and may change our vision of taking care of patients with NSCLC. In conclusion, it seems that mAbs therapy in NSCLC clearly marks the start of a new era in NSCLC treatment, with promises in improving patient survival and quality of life.

Chapter 2 - Lung cancer is one of the most common cancers and non-small cell lung cancer (NSCLC) accounts for 80-85% of lung cancers. There are three main histological subtypes of NSCLC, adenocarcinoma (AD), squamous cell carcinoma (SCC) and large cell carcinoma (LCC), with a difference in survival rate between stage I and II. In addition, AD and SCC respond differently to certain treatments. The prognosis of NSCLC remains poor across all stages, despite advances in staging techniques and treatments. Emerging genomic technologies, especially high-throughput microarray studies, have shown potential in refining current NSCLC diagnosis, classification, prognosis and treatment approaches. Of 90 % of transcribed eukaryotic genomes, only 1-2 % encode for proteins, with the vast majority being non-coding RNAs (ncRNAs). ncRNAs are functional transcripts that do not code for proteins. They are predominantly composed of small double-stranded RNAs (dsRNAs) and are important regulators of gene expression in many eukaryotes. Three types of naturally occurring small RNAs have been described based on their origin or function: short interfering RNAs (siRNAs), repeat-associated short interfering RNAs (rasiRNAs) and microRNAs (miRNAs). Genome-wide profiling has shown that ncRNAs have distinct signatures specific for a certain cancer type. miRNAs are the most widely studied and characterized of all the ncRNAs. It is estimated that there could be as many as a thousand miRNAs, thought to regulate 30-90 % of genes within the human genome. Expression profiling of many microRNAs (miRNAs) in various normal and disease tissues has demonstrated unique spatial and temporal expression patterns. Moreover, global mean expression profiling in several studies has demonstrated differential expression of panels of miRNAs between AD and SCC, suggesting that they may be useful biomarkers for accurate classification of NSCLC. We will outline current knowledge about some specific ncRNAs and their predicted target genes in NSCLC and evaluate their potential as circulating biomarkers and therapeutic targets in NSCLC.

Serum miRNAs distinguish tumours from normal lung tissues and define the histology, growth rate and clinical outcome. Sputum can be used with highly sensitive and specific non-invasive markers for early detection of lung AD. miRNAs could play an important role in the design of innovative therapies for NSCLC. Studies have documented the implications of miRNAs in nearly all carcinogenesis processes. It has also been shown that miRNAs can be delivered systematically and can reduce invasion, proliferation and growth, as well as induce radiosensitivity and resistance. Combining information on ncRNAs with that on other types of biomarkers can improve cancer risk assessment, detection and prognosis of NSCLC.

Chapter 3 - Lung cancer is the leading cause of cancer death in the United States and worldwide. Treatment strategies and options have expanded greatly in recent years, including the use of molecular targeted agents. Targeted therapies, exploiting cancer specific genetic "driver" mutations, while very powerful, are unfortunately limited to subsets of the overall population. In this chapter, the authors will review recent developments of novel therapeutic approach through epigenetic alteration. Epigenetic modification was first discovered by understanding inherited imprinting disorders. Since the discovery of the role of epigenetics in cancer, major strides in deciphering the biology of epigenetic machinery have been made, including DNA methylation, histone acetylation and dynamic alteration of nucleosomal remodeling during the cell cycle. These changes occur early during tumorigenesis as seen in many solid tumors. Biomarkers utilizing abnormal epigenetic signatures are being evaluated for early cancer detection of preneoplastic and preinvasive lesions. In addition, since epigenetic alterations are potentially reversible, as opposed to irreversible genetic alterations (such as insertions, deletions, point mutations and translocations), they offer potential targets for cancer therapy. Epigenetic modulations through DNA methylation and histone deacetylase (HDAC) inhibitors are only beginning to be explored in the clinical setting. Given the almost universal finding of epigenetic alterations in lung cancer, translation of basic epigenomic research into the development of novel agents will provide a new perspective for lung cancer treatments.

Chapter 4 - After a period of stagnation in lung cancer therapeutics, a remarkable molecular revolution occurred in mid-2000's. Molecular characterization of lung carcinoma coincided with the development, and utilization of targeted therapeutic agents. The discovery of EGFR led the movement: after some false starts (INTACT1 and 2), small molecule tyrosine kinase inhibitors gefitinib and then erlotinib gained FDA-approval. Basic science hypotheses of oncogene addition and the discovery of activating mutations has rapidly transitioned from bench to bedside, resulting in a recommendation for up-front testing of lung cancer patients, and the use of targeted agents as first line therapy. Subsequent drug-target pairs followed, such as crizotinib-ALK-EML rearrangements, and in this case the clinical use approval was followed within days by a separate companion diagnostic, underscoring the need for rethinking of the regulatory review and approval paradigm. At this time, a queue of oncogene targets is forming, and inhibitors are being tested in clinical trials with some success: ROS1, RET, C-Met, and BRAF are among them, although others like KRAS remain difficult to target effectively. Regardless of the molecular target, lesional tissue is required for any analysis, and in this process the diagnosis by a pathologist remains the primary step. The challenge arises as the low morbidity means of tissue procurement result in ever smaller amounts of material, while the numbers and variety of assay platforms necessary to match drugs to targets increases. Given this paradigm only a multiplexed approach is feasible, which consequently enforces a common assay platform. Mutational profiling, such as SNaPshot, which captures all known abnormalities should find its way into regular diagnostic practice, and be included in the planning of all lung cancer trials involving new targeted agents.

Chapter 5 – Lung cancer is the leading cause of cancer mortality in both men and women. The majority of these patients present with non-small cell lung cancer (85%) and approximately 45% have locally advanced, stage III disease. Until the 1990s, radiation therapy alone was considered the standard treatment for patients with locally advanced, unresectable disease with median survival times of 10-12 months and 5-year survival rates of 5%. In the early 1990s, several randomized clinical trials showed a survival benefit when platinum-based chemotherapy was delivered concurrently with radiation therapy (RT), with median survival times of 16-17 months and 5-year survival rates of 20-30%. Concurrent chemo-radiation therapy thus became the new standard of care for patients with unresectable stage III disease.

Despite the improved survival outcomes, loco-regional recurrences still remain a problem. Based on radiation oncology first principles, it is felt that higher doses of radiation (up to 100 Gy) may be necessary to adequately control non-small cell lung cancers. Historically, however, doses of radiation therapy had been limited to approximately 60 Gy due to normal tissue dose tolerances and the risks of toxicities to the lung and surrounding tissues. With more modern radiation therapy techniques, such as intensity modulated radiation therapy (IMRT), the incorporation of PET, and 4-D CT treatment planning scans, the role of dose escalation to further improve survival and local control outcomes is being actively evaluated.

Several trials, including the phase I RTOG 0117 study found that higher doses of radiation (up to 74 Gy) could be safely tolerated with concurrent carboplatin and paclitaxel chemotherapy. A follow-up Phase II study demonstrated a survival benefit with this regimen with a median survival time of 21.6 months. Based on these promising results, a randomized phase III trial, RTOG 0617, was initiated comparing carboplatin and paclitaxel chemotherapy with concurrent RT to either 60 Gy or 74 Gy. The interim results of this study were presented at ASTRO 2011 and revealed no survival benefit in the higher dose arm despite similar toxicity profiles between the two groups. These surprising results warrant further evaluation. One hypothesis for the lack of survival benefit is that carboplatin and paclitaxel may represent a suboptimal chemotherapy doublet and that outcomes may be improved if cisplatin-based chemotherapy is given concurrently with increasing doses of radiation therapy. This combination has not yet been tested in clinical trials and is the basis of a current phase I trial at the University of Washington.

Chapter 6 – Non small cell lung cancer (NSCLC)-specific EGFR mutations are the first target for selective treatment identified in NSCLC. The presence of EGFR mutations is a major determinant of tirosine kinase inhibitors (TKIs) response. Most of these “sensitising” mutations include exon 19 deletions, and replacement at exon 21 of leucine 858 by arginine (L858R).

Despite benefits of EGFR TKIs in EGFR-mutant NSCLC, all patients develop progressive tumor growth while receiving treatment, mainly due to the development of resistance, which typically occurs after from 9 to 14 months, depending on the series.

At least 50% of acquired TKI resistance can be attributed to a secondary mutation in the exon 20 of the EGFR gene, the T790M mutation, consisting of the substitution of a methionine residue by a threonine at position 790 of the kinase domain, which arises after exposure to TKIs.

Recently, intermediate and high BRCA1 baseline levels have been described as markers of shorter progression-free survival in patients treated with TKIs.

Other pathways that might explain acquired resistance to EGFR TKIs are the amplification of the MET oncogene (which occurs independently of the T790M mutation in 20% of NSCLC) and the PI3K/Akt, MAPK and NF-KB. The presence of HER2 mutations is also associated with resistance to EGFR TKIs.

In: Non-Small Cell Lung Cancer: New Research
Editor: Lina Pasquariello ISBN: 978-1-62417-804-7

Chapter 1

Therapeutic Antibodies in Non-Small Cell Lung Cancer: An Overview and Future Directions

L. Guilleminault[1,2], E. Lemarié[1,2] and N. Heuzé-Vourc'h[1]
[1]CEPR «Centre d'étude des pathologies respiratoires,
INSERM U1100-EA6305, Université François Rabelais, Tours, France
[2]Service de Pneumologie, CHRU Tours, Tours, France

Abstract

Lung cancer is the leading cause of cancer-related deaths in industrialized countries and non small cell lung cancer (NSCLC) accounts for 85% of all lung cancers. Cisplatin doublet based chemotherapy, which is recommended regimen in first line therapy in advanced or metastatic NSCLC, improves survival but in low proportion. Monoclonal antibodies (mAbs) are a novel promising therapy class used with great results in inflammatory diseases such as rheumatoid arthritis. Antibodies are natural proteins with modular structure, specific pharmacodynamics and pharmacokinetics and possibly produced against any antigens, thus giving them several advantages over small drug therapeutics. In solid tumors, therapeutic mAbs improved progression free survival (PFS) and overall survival (OS) of patients with breast and colon cancers and had considerably changed the treatment in clinical practice. In NSCLC, bevacizumab, an anti-VEGF mAb and cetuximab, an anti-EGFR mAb, are the most studied antibodies. Bevacizumab acts on angiognenesis and improved PFS of non squamous NSCLC but in low proportion as shown in two large phase III trials. It was approved by European Medicines Agency (EMEA) and Food and Drug administration (FDA) as a first line therapy in combination with cisplatin doublet chemotherapy. Cetuximab slightly enhanced OS but did not improve PFS in two large phase III trials. These results added to high adverse effect lead to cetuximab refusal by EMEA and FDA in NSCLC. At first glance, the results of mAbs in NSCLC are somewhat disappointing, in contrast to the benefits obtained with mAb treatments in other solid tumors. However, many other mAbs directed against novel targets, such as IGF1-R or CTLA-4, and new mAbs targeting VEGFR and EGFR pathways with different pharmacodymamical and pharmacokinetic properties are under evaluation and may change our vision of taking care of patients with NSCLC. In conclusion, it seems that mAbs therapy in NSCLC clearly marks the start of a new era in NSCLC treatment, with promises in improving patient survival and quality of life.

Introduction

Cytotoxic agents and radiation therapy have been used to improve the survival and quality of life of patients with cancer, but they no longer increase patient survival and have many side effects. The past few decades have seen huge progress in our understanding of the molecular mechanisms underlying tumor development and dissemination, and this has led to the development of specific therapies with reduced systemic toxicity and improved patient survival. Targeted therapies include small-molecule kinase inhibitors and biotherapeutics. Monoclonal antibodies (mAb) have become major drugs for treating solid and hematological tumors. Antibodies are natural proteins that bind to one of a huge variety of molecular targets with great specificity. Their structure is multimodular, and each domain has a well-defined function. Therapeutic mAbs are not only specific, they also have pharmacodynamical and pharmacokinetic advantages over small molecule drugs, together with limited toxicity. This is why therapeutic mAbs are one of the fastest growing areas of the pharmacological /biotechnological industry, with applications in oncology and in immune and inflammatory disorders. Six therapeutic mAbs have now been approved by the US Food and Drug Administration (FDA) for treating solid tumors, whereas only one was available ten years ago. Lung cancer is the leading cause of cancer fatalities in industrialized countries and non small cell lung cancer (NSCLC) accounts for 85% of all lung cancers. The American Society of Clinical Oncology recommends cisplatin doublet based chemotherapy as the first-line treatment for NSCLC, but the increase in median survival time is modest (Azzoli et al., 2011). Spiro et al. showed that the median survival time of patients with advanced NSCLC treated with cisplatin doublet based chemotherapy (8 months) was only 9 weeks longer than for patients given the best supportive care (5.7 months) (Spiro et al., 2004). Treatment with mAbs has greatly prolonged the survival of patients with solid tumors like breast cancer and colon cancer (Slamon et al., 2001; Hurwitz et al., 2004). They are therefore providing hope to patients with metastatic or locally advanced NSCLC who cannot be treated by surgery. Only one therapeutic antibody, bevacizumab targeting VEGF, is presently approved for treating NSCLC, but several others are under clinical investigation and may improve the survival and quality of life of NSCLC patients. The first part of this chapter summarizes the characteristics of therapeutic antibodies, including their structure, pharmacokinetics, pharmacodynamics and immunogenicity. The second part discusses the details and clinical trials of mAbs designed to treat NSCLC.

1. Therapeutic Antibodies in Cancer: Rationale

Monoclonal antibodies have several pharmacological advantages over small (non-biological) molecules. First, their range of targets is almost limitless. Second, they are highly specific for their targets and so selective that they are unlikely to have unexpected side-effects. Third, there is little risk of them being converted to toxic metabolites. Hence, preclinical and clinical trials tend to be very successful. Last, their pharmacokinetics means that they persist for a long time in the body.

1.1. Structure of Monoclonal Antibodies (Mab)

Antibodies are immunoglobulins (Ig) that are naturally produced by the bodies of humans and other mammals. Human Igs are heterodimeric proteins that can be monomeric or polymeric. Ig monomers are composed of two light (L) chains (25 kDa) and two heavy (H) chains (55 kDa) laid out in a Y-shape. Each chain is made up of modules or domains (Figure 1). Thus, heavy chains start with a variable amino acid sequence (V_H domain) at the tip of the Y-shaped complex, followed by the first constant (C_{H1}) domain. Some classes of Igs then have a hinge region, and there are two or three further C_H domains.

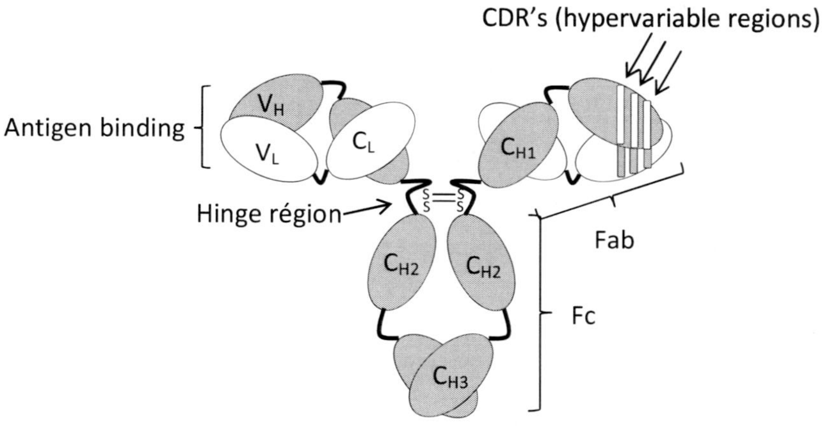

Figure 1. Structure of Ig. Variable light chain (V_L); Variable heavy chain (V_H); constant light chain (C_L); constant heavy chain (C_H); crystallizable fragment (Fc); antigen binding fragment (Fab); hypervariable complementarity-determining regions (CDR).

The two identical heavy chains are joined by disulfide bonds at the hinge region or at the second C_H domain. The light chains have a variable (V_L) domain at the top of the Y-shape complex and a constant (C_L) domain bound by disulphide bonds to the first C_H domain of one of the heavy chains. The light chains interact with the amino-terminal part of the heavy chains to form the Fab domain (fragment of antigen binding) and the carboxyl termini of the heavy chains combine to form the stem or Fc domain (for constant fragment). The two pairs of variable domain (V_L +V_H) at the tip of the Y form the antigen binding site region, which contains three hypervariable complementarity-determining regions (CDR) that define the specific epitope structure that is recognized by the antibody and confer antigen specificity. Monoclonal antibodies, as opposed to polyclonal ones, are antibodies produced by clones of a single B-cell, activated by a single antigen, so that they all bind to a single epitope.

The Fc region corresponds to the effector domain that enables an antibody to interact with molecules such as complement or Fc receptors. Humans produce five classes of Igs that differ by the sequence of their heavy chain constant regions: IgM, IgD, IgG, IgE and IgA. IgA and IgM can form multimers whereas IgG, IgD and IgE are monomeric. IgM and IgD are the first classes of antibodies produced by a B-cell and are implicated in adaptive immunity. They are anchored to the surface of the B cell and are associated with specialized signaling proteins, like the BcR (B cell receptor), a heterodimer composed of two Ig chains, Igα and Igβ. Activated B cells can produce new classes of Ig (IgA, IgE and IgG) that are secreted by the cell, so that they can bind to target antigens outside the cell. IgAs are produced in the lumen of organs like the lungs, intestine, and genitalia. They play a key role in mucosa immunity and IgEs are implicated in immunity to parasites and allergic reactions. IgGs are the most common antibodies secreted by activated human B-cells and thus the main immunoglobulin in the human body. An IgG bound to its antigen can recruit other immune cells and components of the complement system to the antigen reaction site. There are four subclasses of IgGs (IgG1, IgG2, IgG3 and IgG4) that are distinguished by their different heavy chain constant domains and hinge regions. Most monoclonal antibodies (mAb) used as therapeutics are full length IgGs, often of the IgG1 or IgG3 subclasses. Intact IgGs have a molecular weight of ~150 kDa and a valence of 2, which means that each molecule can bind two identical epitopes of the antigen, through the antigen binding domains. Smaller structures derived from IgGs, containing an antigen binding domain (Fab) or a single chain variable fragment (scFv), have also been engineered. Their pharmacokinetics, distributions and pharmacological properties are different from those of intact IgGs (Stockwin and Holmes, 2003).

1.2. History of Therapeutic mAbs

Paul Erhlich was the first to consider antibodies as therapeutics in his "magic bullet" theory in 1908. Achievement of this concept became possible with the development of mouse hybridoma technology by Köhler and Milstein (1975), the first reliable source of monoclonal antibodies (Kohler and Milstein 1975). Despite the fact that they had overcome major technological problems that led to the subsequent development of mAbs for therapeutic use, clinical studies were disappointing. This was because the mouse mAb that were used had a short half-life in human serum and triggered immune responses in human subjects that limited thepossibilites of repeated injections (Shawler et al. 1985; Getts et al. 2010). The human anti-mouse antibody responses (HAMA) was reduced by engineering mAbs that lacked most of the murine sequences, leading to chimeric mAbs containing mouse variable domains fused to human constant regions (Boulianne et al. 1984) and humanized mAbs with murine CDRs grafted into a human IgG backbone (Jones et al. 1986; Kim et al, 2005; Winter et Harris, 1993). In terms of immunogenicity, Hwang and Foote (2005) reported a significant decrease in marked anti-antibody response (AAR) when the Fc regions of murine mAbs were replaced with human sequences. As a result, chimeric and humanized mAbs dominate the antibody-based therapeutics approved for treating humans, while murine monoclonal antibodies (mAbs) have proven useful in diagnostics. Fully human mAbs have been produced recently by transgenic animals or phage display technology and they are being used more and more in clinical trials. However, the improved safety of fully human mAbs is still being debated (Getts et al. 2010). Getts et al. recently reviewed the clinical data for 38 human(ized) and 43 rodent-derived antibodies with contrasting indications and suggest that both types of mAbs trigger similar acute phase reactions and infusion reactions.

Table 1. Therapeutic antibodies approved by the US Food and Drug Administration

Antibody (INN)	Brand name	Approval date	Type	Target	Indication
Abciximab	Reopro	1994	chimeric	Glycoprotein IIb/IIIa	Cardiovascular disease
Adalimumab	Humira	2002	Human	TNF-α	Several auto-immune disease
Alemtuzumab	Campath	2001	Humanized	CD52	Chronic lymphocytoc leukemia
Basiliximab	Simulect	1998	chimeric	IL-2Rα (CD25)	Transplant rejection
Belimumab	Benlysta	2011	Human	B-Cell activating factor	Systemic lupus erythematous
Bevacizumab	Avastin	2004	Humanized	VEGF	Colorectal cancer, age related macular degeneration
Brentuximab	Adcetris	2011	Chimeric	CD30	Anaplastic large cell lymphoma (ALCL) and Hodgkin lymphoma
Canakinumab	Ilaris	2009	Human	IL-1β	Cryopyrin-associated periodic syndromes (CAPS)
Cetuximab	Erbitux	2004	Chimeric	EGFR	Colorectal cancer, Head and neck cancer
Certolizumab	Cimzia	2008	Humanized	TNF-α	Crohn's disease
Daclizumab	Zenapax	1997	Humanized	IL-2Rα receptor (CD25)	Transplant rejection
Denosumab	Prolia, Xgeva	2010	Human	RANK Ligand	Postmenopausal osteoporosis, Solid tumor`s bony metasteses
Eculizumab	Soliris	2007	Humanized	Complement protein C5	Paroxysmal nocturnal hemoglobinuria
Efalizumab	Raptiva	2002	Humanized	CD11a	Psoriasis
Gemtuzumab	Mylotarg	2000	Humanized	CD33	Acute myelogenous leukemia (with calicheamicin)
Golimumab	Simponi	2009	Human	TNF-α	Rheumatoid arthritis, Psoriatic arthritis, and Ankylosing spondylitis
Ibritumomab	Zevalin	2002	murine	CD20	Non-Hodgkin lymphoma (with yttrium-90 or indium-111)
Infliximab	Remicade	1998	Chimeric	TNF-α	Several autoimmune disorders
Ipilimumab	Yervoy	2011	Human	CTLA-4	Melanoma
Muromomab-CD3	Orthoclone OKT3	1986	Murine	T cell CD3 Receptor	Transplant rejection
Natalizumab	Tysabri	2006	Humanized	alpha-4 (α4) integrin	Multiple sclerosis and Crohn's disease
Ofatumumab	Arzerra	2009	Human	CD20	Chronic lymphocytic leukemia
Omalizumab	Xolair	2004	Humanized	IgE	severe allergy-related asthma
Palivizumab	Synagis	1998	Humanized	RSV F protein	Respiratory Syncytial Virus
Panitumumab	Vectibix	2006	Human	EGFR	Colorectal cancer
Ranibizumab	Lucentis	2006	Humanized	VEGF-A	Macular degeneration
Rituximab	Rituxan, Mabthera	1997	Chimeric	CD20	Non-Hodgkin lymphoma

Table 1. (Continued)

Antibody (INN)	Brand name	Approval date	Type	Target	Indication
Tocilizumab (or Atilizumab)	Actemra, RoActemra	2010	Humanized	Anti-IL-6R	Rheumatoid arthritis
Tositumomab	Bexxar	2003	Murine	CD20	Non-Hodgkin lymphoma
Trastuzumab	Herceptin	1998	Humanized	ErbB2/HER-2	Breast cancer

A total of 30 monoclonal antibodies and three fragments are presently approved for sale around the world for treating human diseases and there are nearly 350 candidate mAbs in the pipeline. Several have achieved 'blockbuster' status, with annual sales of over $1 billion. The majority of mAbs on the market or in clinical development are approved or evaluated as treatments for cancer or immunological diseases. Other indications include infectious and central nervous system diseases (Reichert, 2012).

The International Nonproprietary Names (INN) of therapeutic mAbs ends in -mab. The INN of a mAb contains a pre-stem that depends on its origin: "o" for murine antibody, "xi" for chimeric antibody, "zi" for humanized and "u" for fully human antibody.

The approved antibody-based therapeutics listed below illustrates the technologies that have already made it to market.

1.3. Pharmacodynamic

The mechanisms by which therapeutic mAbs act depend on their Fab and/or Fc domains and/or the cytotoxic agents conjugated to them (for summary, see Table 3).

1.3.1. Fab Domain

Therapeutic mAbs bind to their antigen through the Fab domain, usually with high affinity, specificity and selectivity (Nissim and Chernajovsky, 2008; Green et al, 2000; Kim et al, 2005; Ross et al, 2003). The binding of mAbs to antigens has several direct effects, neutralizing infectious agents (palivizumab), sequestrating mediators such as VEGF (bevacizumab) and interfering with receptor interactions, thus disrupting or triggering intracellular transduction cascades.

Engineering mAbs to improve their affinity for their antigen was a very active research area for some time, but increased affinity does not always lead to better pharmacology and in many cases there is an affinity limit. In fact, increasing the affinity of an antitumor mAb may result in limited drug penetration and enhanced adverse side effects due to the mAb binding to normal tissues bearing low concentrations of the targeted antigen.

1.3.2. Fc Domain

Therapeutic antibodies may also act through their Fc domains (Kaneko and Niwa, 2011; Gelderman et al, 2004; Nissim and Chernajovsky, 2008). An IgG bound to its target antigen can be recognized by specific Fc-receptors, FcγRs, which in turn can lead to the recruitment of immune cells effectors, such as natural killer (NK) cells, granulocytes, monocytes or macrophages. This cascade leads to phagocytosis and antibody-dependent cellular cytotoxicity (ADCC). ADCC is an important mechanism by which therapeutic antibodies like rituximab, trastuzumab and cetuximab exert their clinical action. There are three main types of FcγRs for IgG that induce ADCC (FcγRI, FcγRII and FcγRIII) that differ in their affinity for one or more IgG subclass (Table 2) and in their cellular distribution. For example, FcγRIIIa triggers ADCC mainly by NK cells. The clinical relevance of FcγRIIIa is now widely accepted because of the relationship between the functional polymorphism of the receptor and the clinical response of patients to several mAbs, such as rituximab (Cartron et al, 2002 et 2011; Kaneko et Niwa, 2011).

But mAb can also activate the complement system. Antigen-bound antibodies can interact with C1q, leading to complement-dependent cytotoxicity (CDC) (Gelderman et al, 2004; Cartron et al, 2011). Briefly, the binding of the antigen-antibody complex to C1q triggers a proteolytic cascade that results in the formation of bound C3- (C3b) and C5-convertases, and ultimately to the cytolytic membrane attack (MAC) that kills cells bearing the target antigen by disrupting their membranes. The products of C3b proteolysis can also promote complement-receptor enhanced ADCC (CR3-ADCC) by binding to complement receptors (CR3) on granulocytes, macrophages and NK cells and inducing cell-mediated lysis. Activation of the complement cytolytic cascade also depends on the IgG subclass; IgG4 cannot activate complement because of its structure (Table 2). Most of the approved mAb can induce CDC *in vitro*, but the clinical relevance of this function remained unclear for a long time, with only indirect presumptions. However, recent results seem to support the importance of CDC in the clinical outcomes of therapeutic mAbs.

Table 2. Biological activities of human IgGs

Subclass	ADCC	Activation of classical complement pathway
IgG1	++	+
IgG2	+/-	+/-
IgG3	++	++
IgG4	+	-

The results of clinical trials with of atumumab, an optimized anti-CD20 mAb with very potent CDC activity *in vitro,* have been very good. Moreover, Cartron et al have shown that a polymorphism in the CD11b region that interacts with the C3b metabolite to trigger CR3-ADCC influenced the progression-free survival of follicular lymphoma patients given rituximab (Cartron et al, 2011).

Because the therapeutic efficacy of a mAb depends on its antigen binding ability as well as on its capacity to trigger effector functions, investigations have focused on mapping mAbs to determine the residues/structures responsible for these effects and developing strategies to improve mAb-dependent ADCC/CDC by protein engineering or selection/screening (Kim et al., 2005; Kaneko et Niwa, 2011). In particular, it was shown that Fc glycosylation is crucial for the interaction of a mAb with FcγR and that removal of the fucose moiety from the core of the N-glycan enhanced FcγR-dependent ADCC.

1.3.3. Conjugated or Armed mAbs

Therapeutic mAbs, in particular anticancer mAbs, may also act through a conjugated cytotoxic agent (Goldenberg, 2002; Ross et al, 2003; Green et al, 2000). In this case, the mAb acts as a delivery vehicle, carrying the cytotoxic drug to the therapeutic site. Various toxic substances have been combined with mAbs to increase their potency. Radioisotopes are particularly important (radioimmunotherapy) as, in theory, the combination of mAb and radioisotope should deliver focused doses of radiation to the tumor site (Pouget et al, 2011). The death of the targeted cells is due to self-irradiation and that of surrounding tumor cells to bystander effects and cross-fire irradiation. The most widely used radionuclides are β-emitters like ^{131}I, ^{90}Y, and ^{67}Cu that emit low-linear energy transfer (LET) radiation but penetrate tissues deeply (>1μm). In contrast, emitters of α-particles (^{213}Bi, ^{211}At, ^{225}Ac, etc) produce high LET radiation that penetrates tissues poorly. The FDA has approved ibritumomab tiuxetan, an anti-CD20 mAb conjugated to ^{90}Y (in 2002) and ^{131}I-labeled tositumomab, also an anti-CD20 (in 2003), for the treatment of B cell non-Hodgkin's lymphoma.

Other small chemotherapeutic molecules, such as doxorubicin or calichaemicin, are commonly conjugated to mAbs. This may improve the efficacy of these small drugs and limit their toxicity for the target organ. The only mAb in this category that has been approved is gemtuzumab ozogamicin, a humanized anti-CD33 mAb conjugated to the DNA-damaging antibiotic, chalichaemicin. Toxins, such as plant-derived ricin and bacterial-derived *Pseudomonas* exotoxin A, have also been combined with mAbs, but toxins can only act if they are taken up by the target cells.

Interest has increased recently in the possibility of fusing mAb or antibody fragments to cytokines. These fusion proteins, also called immunocytokines, have produced promising results in various experimental models of cancers, auto-immune (psoriasis) and inflammatory (arthritis, endometriosis) diseases and in some clinical trials (Pasche and Neri, 2012). The selective delivery of a cytokine to a disease site by a mAb may increase its therapeutic index and enhance immunomodulation without the toxicity associated with the systemic administration of the cytokine. The choice of cytokines depends on the disease.

Table 3. Multi-faceted activity of therapeutic mAbs

Mechanisms of action
Naked antibody – direct effects Neutralizing infectious agents Interfering with ligand-receptor interactions (antagonist activity) Receptor cross-linking (agonist activity) Sequestrating soluble mediators Antibody as immunogens (anti-idiotype)
Naked antibody – indirect effects Antibody-dependent cellular cytotoxicity (ADCC) Complement-dependent cytotoxicity (CDC)
Armed antibody Delivery of cytotoxic molecules (radionuclides, small chemotherapeutic drugs, toxins...) Immunomodulation (cytokine)

The fused cytokines used to treat cancers are usually IL-2, TNF-α and IFN-γ, whereas anti-inflammatory cytokines, like IL-10, are typically used for chronic diseases.

1.4. Pharmacokinetics of mAbs

Therapeutic antibodies differ from small molecule drugs in their pharmacological properties and also in their pharmacokinetic (PK) profiles. The PK describes the outcome of injecting mAbs into the human body and is a critical parameter in describing their clinical actions. Various factors may contribute to the removal of a mAb, including the amount of the target antigen, immune reactions to the antibody, the delivery route and patient characteristics (Keizer et al., 2010; Paintaud, 2009, Wang et al., 2008). One of these factors, the FcRn receptor, plays a critical role regulating mAb pharmacokinetics (Kuo et al, 2010; Rojas and Apodaca, 2002; Ward and Ober, 2009; Tesar and Björkman, 2010).

1.4.1. FcRn Receptor

The FcRn, also known as the Brambell receptor, is a major histocompatibility complex (MHC) class I-like molecule and a member of the FcγR, which binds both albumin and IgG via their Fc domain. FcRn is a heterodimer composed of a 50 kDa transmembrane α-chain that is noncovalently associated with a β2-microglobulin (15 kDa). The receptor is expressed by cells of the vascular endothelium, of various polarized epithelia and by hematopoietic cells (Kuo et al., 2010; Rojas and Apodaca, 2002; Ward and Ober, 2009; Tesar and Björkman, 2010). The binding of antibodies to FcRn is pH dependent, occurring at slightly acidic pH (6.0-6.5). FcRn receptors at the apical surface of cells in an acidic environment like the intestine lumen bind IgG molecules, transport them to the basolateral surface where the pH is closer to neutrality and release them. FcRn can also take up IgG after pinocytosis or endocytosis into acidified endosomes. The IgG molecules bound to FcRn in endosomes escape proteolytic degradation by the lysosome and are either recycled to the apical plasma membrane or delivered by transcytosis to the basolateral part of the cells where the neutral pH favours the dissociation of IgG from FcRn.

Thus the FcRn protect IgGs from catabolism and mediates the transport of IgG across epithelial/endothelial cells. Recent studies have also shown that it is involved in antigen presentation by professional antigen-presenting cells. It therefore plays a central role in the absorption and distribution of mAbs from the bloodstream to the tissues, and strongly influences their half-life in biological fluids.

1.4.2. Administration and Absorption

The majority of marketed mAbs are delivered via the intravenous (iv) route, which ensures rapid and complete systemic exposure to the mAb. However, several approved mAb are also administered extravascularly, either subcutaneously (sc) (adalimumab, omalizumab, etc) or intramuscularly (im) (palivizumab). As monoclonal antibodies are large molecules, their absorption may be facilitated by the lymphatic system following sc or im delivery. In this case, they are usually absorbed slowly, so that it generally takes a few days for the peak plasma concentration to be reached, and they are often less bioavailable than small molecules. Wang et al. studied transgenic animals that were KO for FcRn and showed that FcRn receptors may contribute to the absorption of mAbs delivered sc (Wang et al, 2008).

Our group has also investigated the pulmonary route for the local delivery of mAbs to the lungs (Maillet et al., 2011), but this delivery route is not yet used for the clinical delivery of mAbs.

1.4.3. Distribution

Their size and hydrophilic nature mean that mAbs do not readily cross the vascular endothelium by passive diffusion (Wang et al, 2008; Keizer et al, 2010). The extravasation of mAbs from the blood into the peripheral tissues occurs mainly by convection and/or transcytosis via the FcRn. Consequently, the concentration of unbound mAb in most tissues is ten times lower than in the bloodstream (Paintaud, 2009).

Their large size and their high affinity for their antigen often limit the distribution of mAbs within targeted tissues, resulting in a low distribution volume (Rudnick et al., 2011). This slow escape from the systemic system into solid tumors and the small distribution volume results in their poor, heterogeneous tumor penetration, which may hamper their therapeutic action. This is the primary rationale for delivering radiolabeled mAb in fractionated doses instead of a single dose, and for investigating local delivery routes to increase the exposure of the target organ to mAbs (Keizer et al., 2011; Maillet et al., 2008 and 2011).

Smaller antibody fragments may cross the endothelium and penetrate into the peripheral tissues more easily, thus overcoming the poor distribution of intact mAbs.

1.4.4. Metabolism and Elimination

Monoclonal antibodies are metabolized to peptides or amino acids that can be recycled for the *de novo* synthesis of proteins, or excreted by the kidneys. Thus, mAb are metabolised in various tissues and the blood and several elimination mechanisms are involved. First, mAbs may be eliminated by intracellular proteolysis inthe liver, the reticuloendothelial system, including the phagocytic cells of the immune system, and cells bearing the targeted antigen. Antigen-bound mAbs bound to FcγR (I to III) or mAbs bound to their antigen on the cell surface can be internalized and then broken down in the lysosomes. Also, mAbs may be engulfed by the plasma membrane and taken into cells by fluid-phase pinocytosis or endocytosis. FcRn is associated with mAbs in acidic endosomes and protects them from proteolytic degradation. FcRn then recycles or transports them across cells and releases them at the cell surface. FcRn protect IgGs from catabolism in endothelial cells, and recycle them, thereby regulating the amount of IgG in the blood plasma. The saturable nature of the interaction of FcRn with IgG governs the concentration of endogenous IgGs in the plasma. When the IgG concentration is low, most of it is bound to FcRn, and it is either recycled or transported from the apical to the basolateral surface of the endothelial cells. But when the IgG concentration is high, all the FcRn molecules in endosomes are saturated. Any the remaining unbound IgG is delivered to the lysosomes, where it is destroyed by intracellular proteinases (Rojas and Apodaca, 2002; Kuo et al., 2010; Ward and Ober, 2009; Tesar and Björkman, 2010). Because mAbs are usually administered at doses of 10mg/kg, which is the average plasma concentration of endogenous IgG, therapeutic doses of mAbs do not generally saturate FcRn recycling (Wang et al, 2008; Keizer et al, 2010).

1.4.5. Engineered IgG and Their Pharmacokinetics

One major advantage of mAb over small therapeutic molecules is that IgGs remain in a patient's circulation much longer. The unique ability of FcRn to prolong the half-life of IgG in biological fluids and promote their transcellular transport has inspired the engineering of novel mAbs whose Fc has been modified to influence the functions of FcRn (Ward and Ober

2009; Kaneko and Niwa, 2011). Although some studies showed a correlation between the enhanced FcRn-binding of engineered IgGs and their longer half-lives *in vivo* and more efficient transport, other studies have not. This may be because of the improved affinity at neutral pH which may limit the release of IgG during exocytosis.

Although engineering small antibody fragments like scFv and Fab fragments improves their ability to penetrate tissues or tumors, it may also reduce their half-life in the plasma because they no longer interact with FcRn.

1.4.6. Other Factors Influencing the Pharmacokinetics of mAbs

The variation in the way individuals respond to mAbs is attributed to differences in the pharmacokinetics of mAbs in each individual (Paintaud, 2009). Thus, immune reactions and the immunogenicity of mAbs influence the pharmacokinetics of mAbs in patients. It has been suggested that anti-antibody may affect the rates at which mAbs are eliminated, but the published data indicate that it is difficult to predict whether immunization will increase the rate of mAb elimination and influence clinical responses.

Demographic factors, such as body weight and gender also affect the pharmacokinetics of mAbs (Keizer et al., 2010; Paintaud, 2009). The PKs of bevacizumab, rituximab and infliximab are particularly dependent on human gender.

Finally tumor mass also modulates mAb pharmacokinetics. Studies on a murine model of lymphoma expressing human CD20 have shown that the concentration of rituximab in the blood is inversely correlated with tumor mass (Daydé et al, 2009). And the pharmacokinetics of trastuzumab in breast cancer is modulated by the number of metastatic sites.

1.5. Immunogenicity and Safety of mAbs

1.5.1. Anti-Antibody Response (AAR)

The immunogenicity of mAbs refers to their ability to induce an AAR and results from an immune response of a patient to the therapeutic mAb. An AAR is generally attributed to non-human sequences in the therapeutic mAb, and is usually considered to be a negative predictive factor for mAb clinical efficacy (Hwang and Foote, 2005). However, this assumption may be unfounded. Getts et al. found that, while rodent-derived mAbs more frequently triggered an AAR than did other mAbs, the AAR may be correlated with a greater therapeutic efficacy for certain murine mAbs (Getts et al. 2010). Thus, a murine anti-HLA-DR10 mAb (Lym-1) was particularly effective for treating patients with non-Hodgkin lymphoma who had high HAMA titers (Azinovic et al. 2006). This may be attributed to idiotypic anti-Lym-1 antibodies that may also bind to the targeted antigen, thus enhancing tumor destruction via ADCC or CDC. However, the mechanisms underlying the greater efficacy due to HAMA remain to be elucidated.

The immunogenicity of mAbs may also be attributed to the presence of mAb conglomerates in the injected preparation (Nezlin, 2010). Immunoglobulins do not just interact with their antigen and a variety of proteins (Fc receptor, anti-antibodies, etc), they can also interact with each other to form self-aggregates. Dimers, oligomers and even aggregates of mAbs occur through Fab-Fab and Fc-Fc interactions, and other aggregation-prone sites, under conditions such as long-term storage, high concentrations, agitation and low pH. The presence of mAb conglomerates is a critical issue in clinical practice as they may elicit an immunological response and thus reduce the efficacy of the mAb.

1.5.2. Cytokine Release Syndrome (CRS)

Therapeutic mAbs are generally safe (for reviews Brennan et al, 2010; Getts et al, 2010; Hansel et al, 2010). Their high selectivity reduces the potential of non-mechanism-based toxicity and their bioconversion is well-defined. Antibodies are metabolized to non-toxic peptides and amino acids by circulating phagocytic cells or by their target cells. The toxicity of mAbs is mainly associated with excessive pharmacological activity and/or the presence of the targeted antigen in tissues where the therapeutic effect is useless. Serious adverse effects of mAbs include anaphylaxis, a rare response to the first infusion (IgE-mediated), and the cytokine release syndrome (CRS) or cytokine storm (Bugelski et al, 2009; Descotes, 2009). The CRS involves a massive secretion of pro-inflammatory mediators following an acute phase reaction or the pharmacological activity of immunomodulatory mAbs. Several approved therapeutic mAbs of different origins trigger a CRS, including alemtuzumab, muromonab-CD3, rituximab, and tosituzumab. The CRS is usually mild and and self-limiting, with acute phase reactions and it undoubtedly results from the interaction of the mAb-Fc with its receptor. However, a CRS can also be life threatening. When the CD28 superagonist mAb, TGN1412, was given to healthy volunteers in 2006 it induced dramatic severe side effects, including renal failure, severe blood lymphopaenia and monocytopaenia, and acute respiratory distress syndrome. These were not predicted by animal studies.

Overall, the clinical data indicate that the way humans interact with and respond to mAbs varies from one individual to another and seems difficult to predict. Moreover, a "human" mAb is not necessarily safer, less immunogenic, or more effective than any other mAb.

2. Therapeutic Antibodies in Non Small Cell Lung Cancer (NSCLC): Pre-Clinical and Clinical Studies

2.1. Anti-VEGF Antibodies

2.1.1. Vascular Epidermal Growth Factor (VEGF) and NSCLC

Angiognesis has been known to play a role in cancer pathophysiology for over a century (Ferrara et al., 2002; Lewis et al., 1927). VEGF (also called VEGF A) is involved in angiogenesis and belongs to a gene family encoding proteins like placental growth factor (PGF), VEGF B, VEGF C, VEGF D and VEGF E (Senger et al., 1983; Ferrara et al., 2003). VEGF C and D regulate lymphatic angiogenesis (Ferrara et al., 2002; Karkkainen 2002). VEGF-B is found in many tissues, but is particularly abundant in the heart and skeletal muscle (Olofsson et al., 1999). Native VEGF A is a 45 kDa heparin-binding homodimeric glycoprotein that interacts with two related receptors, tyrosine kinase VEGFR-1 and VEGFR-2 (Ferrara et al., 1989). These receptors are present on endothelial cells and hematopoietic cells, and are autophosphorylated once VEGF has become bound to them. Despite the high affinity of VEGF for VEGFR1, the kinase activity of this receptor is weak (Waltenberger et al., 1994). VEGFR1 is essential during development but its signaling remains unclear (Sullivan and Brekken, 2010). VEGFR-2 (or fetal liver kinase-1 (Flk-1)) is the predominant mediator of VEGF-induced angiogenic, mitogenic activities, and permeability signaling (Takahashi et al., 2005). The binding of VEGF to VEGFR2 causes the receptor to dimerize and auto-phosphorylate (Roskoski, 2007). Phosphorylation of the principal residues on VEGFR2, tyrosines 1175 and 1214, triggers signaling cascades implicating PI3K, AKT, PLCγ, p38 MAPK and p42/44 MAPK and the subsequent proliferation, survival and vascular permeability. VEGFR-2 also contributes to the re-organization of the cytoskeleton in these cells via phosphorylation of FAK (focal adhesion kinase) (Gerber et al., 1998; Fujio et al., 1999). The VEGFR-2–mediated proliferation of endothelial cells involves activation of a phospholipase C gamma-protein kinase signaling pathway (Veikkola et al., 2000).

Clinical trials on several tumor systems, including lung cancer, have shown that the overproduction of VEGF is associated with tumor progression and poor prognosis (Fontanini et al., 1997; Kadota et al., 2008). A recent meta-analysis showed that VEGF overproduction, assessed by immunohistochemistry, is associated with poor prognosis with a hazard ratio of 1.46 (1.38–1.55) in NSCLC, 1.46 (1.38–1.54) in stage I–III NSCLC, 1.27 (1.06 –1.47) in adenocarcinoma, 1.57 (1.43–1.70) in stage I NSCLC (Zhan et al., 2009).

2.1.2. Bevacizumab

2.1.2.1. Preclinical Studies with Bevacizumab

Bevacizumab is a recombinant humanized monoclonal antibody directed against soluble VEGF. It is a human IgG1 with a murine hypervariable region (Presta et al., 1997). The high concentrations of VEGF in several tumors led to the proposal of the anti-VEGF antibody, bevacizumab or its murine parent A.4.6.1, as potential cancer treatments. The anti-tumor effects of these anti-VEGF antibodies were assessed in mice. Anti-VEGF antibodies inhibit the growth of a variety of human tumor cell lines in a murine xenograft model (Lee et al., 2000; Pham et al., 1998; Kim et al. 1993). For NSCLC, these antibodies produced the same results in a murine xenograft model with CALU-6 cells, which are derived from a human lung anaplastic carcinoma (Kabbinavar et al., 1995). The hypoxia-induced production of VEGF seems to be important in the resistance of tumors to radiotherapy and chemotherapy (Harmey et al., 2002.) The antibody A.4.6.1 significantly improved the antitumor effects of chemotherapy and radiotherapy (Kabinavar et al., 1995). A combination of radiotherapy and anti-VEGF antibody seems to be synergist. The response of mice with Lewis lung carcinoma, a spontaneous lung tumor of C57BL/6 mice, given the combined treatments was greater than a simple additive anti-tumor effect (Gorsky et al., 1999).

2.1.2.2. Pharmacokinetic

The elimination half-life of bevacizumab in cynomolgus monkeys was 8-10 days, its clearance was 4.76-5.78 ml/day/kg and the time to maximum plasma concentration was 5-33 minutes for doses of 2, 10, 50 mg/kg IV. Its absorption and maximum plasma concentrations were dose-dependent. A recent analysis of 8 large clinical trials to determine its pharmacokinetics in humans foundwed that steady-state peak concentrations were approximately 20% higher with doses of 7.5 mg/kg every 3 weeks (270 lg/mL) than with doses of 5 mg/kg every 2 weeks (215 lg/mL) (Lu et al., 2008). The steady-state average (73 g/mL) and trough concentrations (85.1 g/mL) for the two regimens were similar. The estimated terminal half-life was almost 20 days for both men and women. Body weight and gender were the most significant factors influencing variations in clearance between patients; clearance was 26% faster in men than in women. Clearance was 19% faster in patients with low serum albumin concentrations than in typical patients, and 23% faster in those with high serum alkaline.

2.1.3. Clinical Trials of Bevacizumab Combined with Chemotherapy

2.1.3.1. Phase II Clinical Trial

The main clinical trials with bevacizumab are detailed in table 4. Bevacizumab was first shown to be clinically active against advanced, metastatic or recurrent NSCLC, in the phase II trial AVF0757g (Johnsson et al., 2004). The 99 patients, randomly included in this trial, received either bevacizumab 7.5 mg/kg combined with carboplatin/paclitaxeln (PC) (n=32), or bevacizumab 15 mg/kg combined PC every 3 weeks (n=35). The 32 remaining patients in the control arm were treated with carboplatin and paclitaxel alone. The treatment with carboplatin and paclitaxel plus bevacizumab (15 mg/kg) resulted in a higher response rate (31.5%) than the controls (18.8%), longer median time to progression (7.4 months; controls 4.2 months) and a modest increase in survival (17.7 months; controls 14.9 months). The results for 15 mg/kg bevacizumab were better than those for 7.5 mg/kg. Pulmonary hemorrage was the most severe adverse event, which occurred almost always in squamous carcinomas (4/13 patients) compared to 2/54 patients with adenocarcinomas. The next trials with bevacizumab were therefore done only on patients with non-squamous cell histology and no history of relevant pulmonary hemorrage.

A recent trial showed that the toxicity of bevacizumab associated with carboplatin and gemcitabine is reasonable (only three cases of grade 3 bleeding in 48 patients) (Clement-duchene et al., 2010). The median time to the first event (progression/death/toxicity requiring discontinuation) was 6.4 months and the median overall survival (OS) time was 12.8 months.

It was shown recently that cisplatine plus permetrexed was a particularly efficient treatment for adenocarcinoma and this combination is now the first choice in advanced lung adenocarcinoma (Scagliotti et al., 2008). Bevacizumab was initially considered to be combined with permetrexed in second or third line therapy. In the phase II trial of Suk Heist et al., 36 patients were treated with bevacizumab combined with oxaliplatin and permetrexed (Suk Heist et al., 2008). This uncontrolled study evaluated the tumor responses of 34 patients. None of them had a complete response, nine (27%) had a partial response, the disease was stable in 15 (44%), and the disease progressed in 10 (29%). The median progression-free survival time was 5.8 months and the median overall survival time was 12.5 months. This regimen was reasonably toxic. Another phase II trial on 48 patients with non squamous non small cell lung cancer used bevacizumab combined with permetrexed as the second line treatment (Adjei et al., 2010). Polymorphisms in genes responsible for pemetrexed transport (reduced folate carrier [SLC19A1]) and metabolism (folylpolyglutamate synthase [FPGS] and gamma-glutamyl hydrolase [GGH]) evaluated in germline DNA (blood) were analyzed to see whether these markers were correlated with treatment outcome. The primary endpoint of a 70% success rate was not reached. The median overall survival time was 8.6 months and the progression-free survival time was 4.0 months. Toxicites were acceptable because the most common grade 3 or 4 nonhematological adverse events were fatigue (13%), dyspnea (10%), and thrombosis (10%). The exon 6 (2522)C3T polymorphism in SLC19A1 was significantly correlated with the 3-month progression-free status and with progression free survival. The IVS1(1307)C3T polymorphism in GGH was correlated with the overall survival time.

The cisplatin-permetrexed combination and treatment based on the bevacizumab-cisplatin-gemcitabine trio are two possible first line therapies for non-squamous non small cell lung cancer. Only one study has assessed both these therapies by indirect treatment comparison (Nuijten et al., 2011). The results of two previously published studies were used (Scagliotti et al., 2008; Reck et al., 2009). A hazard ratio of 0.83 for progression-free survival for bevacizumab plus cisplatin and gemcitabine suggested that the risk of disease progression on this treatment is 17% lower that for pemetrexed plus cisplatin. The Markov model used in this study predicted that bevacizumab plus cisplatin and gemcitabine resulted in longer progression-free survival (2.5 months) and overall survival times than did pemetrexed plus cisplatin.

Combinations of 15 mg/kg bevacizumab plus other double chemotherapies were also assessed. One trial treated 99 patients with non small cell lung cancer with bevacizumab combined with oxaliplatin and gemcitabine (Lilenbaum et al., 2008). The median time to progression was 5.5 months, which approached that seen in phase III studies, and the median survival time was 13.7 months. This uncontrolled trial has had little impact on clinical practice. Another trial used bevacizumab combined with carboplatin and docetaxel to treat 40 cases of non squamous non small cell lung cancer; there were high incidences of bleeding (13%) and thromboembolic events (13%) (William et al., 2010). The median progression-free survival time was 7.9 months and the median overall survival time was 16.5 months.

2.1.3.2. Phase II Clinical Trial in Squamous Non Small Cell Lung Cancer

As suggested by the phase II clinical trial conducted by Johnsson et al., using bevacizumab to treat squamous NSCLC could result in a fatal pulmonary hemorrage (Johnsson et al., 2005). Bevacizumab was assessed once again in patients with squamous NSCLC in a recent trial named the BRIDGE study (Hainsworth et al., 2011). Patients with advanced squamous NSCLC and no history of pulmonary hemorrage were given two cycles of carboplatin-paclitaxel as first line therapy followed by 3 to 6 cycles of carboplatin-paclitaxel combined with bevacizumab. Only one (3.2%) of the 31 patients given at least one dose of bevacizumab had a grade 3 pulmonary haemorrhage. Treatment was discontinued and the patient died due to disease progression. The median progression-free survival time was short, 6.2 months. Further studies with more patients are needed to obtain clear evidence for the safety and efficacy of bevacizumab for treating squamous NSCLC.

2.1.3.3. Phase III Clinical Trials in Non Squamous Non Small Cell Lung Cancer

The European approval of bevacizumab as a first-line therapy for advanced or recurrent NSCLC without predominantly squamous cell histology is based on the results of the trials ECOG 4599 and AVAiL (Avastin in Lung) (Sandler et al., 2006; Reck et al. 2009). In both trials, bevacizumab was given together with chemotherapy to patients with advanced or recurrent non-small cell lung cancer; those with squamous carcinomas were excluded. Bevacizumab treatment was continued until the disease progressed. The chemotherapy was cisplatin plus gemcitabine in the European trial (AVAiL), while it was carboplatin plus paclitaxel in the American trial. The patients in both trials were treated with up to 6 cycles.

The most recent ASCO guidelines now state that first-line chemotherapy for patients who are not responding should be stopped at 4 cycles (Pfister et al., 2003.). In the ECOG trial, 444 patients were given double chemotherapy alone and 434 patients received double chemotherapy plus 15 mg/kg bevacizumab. The median survival time of the group given chemotherapy plus bevacizumab was 12.3 months; this was significantly longer than the 10.3 months for the patients given chemotherapy alone-. The median progression-free survival time of the group given bevacizumab was better (6.2 months) than that of the control group (4.5 months). Clinically significant bleeding was more frequent (4.4%) in the patients treated with bevacizumab than in those given chemotherapy alone (0.7%).

Table 4. Main clinical trials of bevacizumab combined with chemotherapy as first or second line therapy in NSCLC. PC: Paclitaxel/Carboplatin, Oxali/Pem: Oaliplatin/Pemetrexed. Oxali/Gem: Oaliplatin/Gemcitabine. CG: Carboplatin/Gemcitabine. CD: Carboplatin/Docetaxel. Pem. Pemetrexed. Cis/Gem: Cisplatin/Gemcitabine. PFS: progression free survival. OS: overall survival

Authors	Drugs	Patients	Response rate	Toxicity
Phase II Johnsson et al., 2004	Arm A: Bevacizumab 7.5 mg/kg + PC Arm : Bevacizumab 15 mg/kg + PC	n=99	PFS : Arm A=7.4 months Arm B=4.2 months OS: Arm A=17.7 months Arm B= 14.9 months	Severe pulmonary hemorrage in squamous carcinoma patients
Phase II Suk Heist et al., 2008	Bevacizumab 15 mg/kg+ Oxali/Pem	n=36	PFS : 5.8 months OS: 12.5 months	1 grade 5 hemoptysis
Phase II Lilenbaum et al., 2008	Bevacizumab 15 mg/kg+ Oxali/Gem	n=44	PFS : 5.5 months OS: 13.7 months	5 hypertension 1 allergic reaction
Phase II Clement-duchene et al, 2010	Bevacizumab 15 mg/kg+CG	n=48	PFS : 6.4 months OS: 12.8 months	high incidences of bleeding and thromboembolic events
Phase II William et al., 2010	Bevacizumab 15 mg/kg+CD	n=40	PFS : 7.9 months OS: 16.5 months	
Phase II Adjei et al., 2010	Bevacizumab 15 mg/kg+ Pem (2nd line)	n=48	PFS : 4 months OS: 8.6 months	
Phase II Hainsworth et al., 2011	Bevacizumab 15 mg/kg+CP (Suqamous NSCLC)	n=31	PFS : 6.2 months	1 Pulmonary hemorrage
Phase III Sandler et al., 2006 (ECOG 4599)	Arm A: Bevacizumab 15 mg/kg+PC Arm B: PC alone	n=818	PFS: Arm A= 12.3 months Arm B= 10.3 months OS: Arm A=6.2 months Arm B=4.5 months	Significant hypertension, proteinuria and bleeding with bevacizumab
Phase III Reck et al., 2009 (AVAiL)	Arm A: Cis/Gem alone Arm B: Bevacizumab 7.5 mg/kg+Cis/Gem Arm C: Bevacizumab 15 mg/kg+Cis/Gem	n=1043	PFS: Arm A= 6.7 months Arm B= 6.5 months Arm C= 6.1 months No sufficient data for OS analysis	Significant hypertension, and bleeding with bevacizumab

The American results were confirmed three years later by the European regimen in AVAil trial. This trial with three arms included 345 patients treated with 7.5 mg/kg bevacizumab plus double chemotherapy, 351 given 15 mg/kg bevacizumab alone and 347 given chemotherapy alone. The progression-free survival time was significantly longer in the two groups treated with bevacizumab (6.7 months on the low dose and 6.5 months for those on the high dose) than for the chemotherapy alone patients (6.1 months). The follow-up was too short for overall survival (OS) analysis, but median survival times were unusually long, over 13 months, for all three patient groups. The grade 3 pulmonary hemorrhage rate was 1.5% for the low dose bevacizumab group, 0.9 for the high dose bevacizumab group, and 0.6 for the control group. Unlike in first study of Johnsson et al., in AVAiL there is no difference between the two doses of bevacizumab.

2.1.3.4. Phase IV Clinical Trials in Non Squamous Non-Small Cell Lung Cancer

The approval of bevacizumab by the FDA and EMEA required a phase IV study to assess its safety in "real life" with unselected patients. Patients with locally advanced, metastatic, or recurrent non-squamous NSCLC were given bevacizumab (7·5 or 15 mg/kg every 3 weeks) plus standard chemotherapy for up to six cycles, followed by bevacizumab alone until disease progression in the SAiL phase 4 single-arm study in Europe (Crino et al., 2010). The primary endpoint was safety. The incidence of clinically significant (grade ≥3) adverse events of special interest among the 2212 patients included was generally low. Thromboembolism occurred in 172 (8%) patients, hypertension in 125 (6%), bleeding in 80 (4%), proteinuria in 67 (3%) and pulmonary haemorrhage in 15 (1%) patients. Fifty seven (3%) patients died because of adverse events. The American phase IV study, the ARIES trial, on 1,970 patients with advanced NSCLC assessed the safety of bevacizumab as a first-line therapy for NSCLC; it was combined with double chemotherapy (Sandomenico et al., 2012). The median progression-free survival time for the whole cohort was 6.7 months and it was 6.8 months for the elderly patients (70 years of age or older). The median progression-free survival time of patients on therapeutic anticoagulant was 6.2 months and their overall survival time was 11.0 months. The median progression-free survival time of patients with a history of haemoptysis was 6.2 months and their overall survival time was 11.6 months. The adverse event rates were also similar for the overall cohort, except for more arterial thromboembolic events in the older patients and in those with poor general status. The incidence of grade 3 to 5 bleeding events in all NSCLC patients was 3.4%.

2.1.3.5. Bevacizumab as Maintenance Therapy: Current Concepts

Maintenance therapy is defined as therapy that is continued without a break after the end of first line therapy. Some authors have suggested improving the efficiency of lung cancer treatment by using a combination of bevacizumab and other treatments as a maintenance therapy. A phase II trial was carried on 50 patients given pemetrexed-carboplatin and 15 mg/kg bevacizumab every 3 weeks for six cycles (Patel et al., 2009a). Pemetrexed and bevacizumab were continued in patients with a response or stable disease until there was disease progression or unacceptable toxicity. Thirty patients (60%) completed six treatment cycles, and nine (18%) completed at least 18 treatment cycles. The median progression-free time for the 49 patients whose response could be assessed was 7.8 months and the overall survival time was 14.1 months. There was no grade 3 or greater hemorrhagic events.

2.1.3.6. Bevacizumab as Maintenance Therapy: Future Directions

The relative good tolerance of bevacizumab in previous trials led to a phase III study (Patel et al., 2009b) on nearly 900 patients with advanced non squamous NSCLC. As part of this ongoing study, they will be given either 4 cycles of pemetrexed/carboplatin/bevacizumab followed by a maintenance phase of pemetrexed/bevacizumab (arm A), or 4 cycles of a combination of paclitaxel/carboplatin/bevacizumab followed by bevacizumab maintenance (arm B). The maintenance therapy will be continued until there is disease progression or the toxic effects become unmanageable. The objectives of this study are to compare the overall survival times and the progression-free survival times of the 2 treatment arms. If the primary objective is achieved, this study will provide robust results and will change clinical practice. Patients in another trial in progress, the ERACLE trial, will be given either an initial treatment with pemetrexed and cisplatin followed by maintenance with pemetrexed or an initial treatment with carboplatin plus paclitaxel plus bevacizumab, followed by maintenance with bevacizumab (Galetta et al. 2011). The primary objective of the study is to compare quality of life of the patients in the treatment arms. A third trial, which is also in progress, is designed to directly compare maintenance therapies that useh bevacizumab or pemetrexed (Zinner et al., 2010). The patients with non squamous NSCLC in this randomized trial will be given pemetrexed/carboplatin followed by maintenance pemetrexed or paclitaxel/carboplatin /bevacizumab, followed by maintenance bevacizumab. The primary end-point is progression-free survival without any grade ≥ 4 toxicity. Finally, the AVAPERL trial will also assess maintenance with bevacizumab, but only preliminary results are available (Bankhead et al., 2011). The patients with non squamous NSCLC taking part in this trial are given pemetrexed/cisplatin/bevacizumab followed by either pemetrexed or pemetrexed /bevacizumab. Preliminary results indicate that pemetrexed/bevacizumab provides better maintenance, with a progression-free survival time of 10.2 months, although patients on bevacizumab maintenance treatment have a progression-free survival time of 6.6 months. The toxicity rates in the two arms seem to be similar.

2.1.4. Clinical trials of bevacizumab combined with targeted therapy

2.1.4.1. Erlotinib

Erlotinib is a HER-1/epidermal growth factor receptor tyrosine kinase inhibitor (TKI) that improves the survival time of patients with advanced NSCLC who have been given one or two prior chemotherapy regimens (Shepherd et al., 2005). Response rate was higher among women, nonsmokers, Asians patients. Administering bevacizumab and erlotinib together may have additional clinical benefits for cancer patients with advanced disease because bevacizumab and erlotinib act on two different pathways, one of which is critical for tumor growth, while the other regulates angiogenesis.

2.1.4.1.1. Phase I and II Trials

As targeted therapies are important anticancer agents, it is essential to use the combination of molecules that provides the best improvement in patient survival.

Bevacizumab has mostly been evaluated in association with oral erlotinib, which is approved for use alone as a second line therapy of NSCLC with no restriction. The phase I/II study by Herbst gave bevacizumab associated with erlotinib to 40 patients (phase I) and 34 (phase II) with non squamous NSCLC (Table 5) (Herbst et al., 2005). The phase I study used 3 increasing doses of bevacizumab, whereas the 34 in the phase II study were given 15 mg/kg bevacizumab every 3 weeks in association with 150 mg/d erlotinib. The most common adverse events were a mild to moderate rash, diarrhoea, and proteinuria. Preliminary data showed no pharmacokinetic interaction between bevacizumab and erlotinib. Only 8 of the phase II patients (20.0%) had a partial response, while the best response of 26 (65.0%) was a stable disease. The progression-free survival for the 34 phase II patients was 6.2 months and the median overall survival time was 12.6 months. A second phase II study on 120 patients with non squamous NSCLC compared bevacizumab combined with either erlotinib or chemotherapy (docetaxel or pemetrexed) to chemotherapy alone (docetaxel or pemetrexed) as a second line therapy (Herbst et al., 2007). The few adverse events that did occur were similarly frequent in all three groups. Fewer patients (13%) in the bevacizumab-erlotinib arm discontinued treatment as a result of adverse events than in the chemotherapy alone (24%) or bevacizumab-chemotherapy (28%) arms. Pulmonary haemorrhage occurred in 2 of the 39 patients treated with bevacizumab and chemotherapy, in 1 of the 39 given bevacizumab and erlotinib, and in none of the 42 treated with chemotherapy alone. Although not statistically significant, the risk of disease progression or death seemed to be lower among patients treated with bevacizumab-chemotherapy and with bevacizumab-erlotinib than in those treated with chemotherapy alone. The progression-free survival time was 3 months for those treated with chemotherapy alone, 4.4 months for those given bevacizumab-chemotherapy, and 4.8 months for patients given bevacizumab-erlotinib. The overall survival time was 8.6 for patients given chemotherapy alone, 12.6 months for those given bevacizumab-chemotherapy, and 13.7 months for those treated with bevacizumab-erlotinib. A more recent phase II study on 47 chemonaive patients with non squamous NSCLC used 15 mg/kg bevacizumab combined with erlotinib 150 mg/d until progression, including molecular imaging (Dingemans et al., 2011). The tumor response was measured by computed tomography, 2-[fluorine-18]fluoro-2-deoxy-D-glucose (FDG–PET) and dynamic contrast-enhanced magnetic resonance imaging (DCE-MRI). The median progression-free survival (PFS) time was 3.8 months and the median overall survival (OS) time was 6.9 months. Grade 3/4 toxicity was generally rare. The presence of KRAS (n = 10) or EGFR mutations (n = 5) did not influence outcome. There was a >20% decrease in standard uptake after 3 weeks of treatment, as measured by positron emission tomography, which predicted a longer progression-free survival time (9.7 months) and a >40% decrease in Ktrans, as assessed by DCE-MRI, which did not predict a longer PFS time. The overall survival time was surprisingly low in this study, but the early response evaluation by FDG–PET seemed to be the best predictor of progression-free survival. Another phase II single arm-study is currently under way to assess bevacizumab-erlotinib as second or third line therapy (Tanaka et al., 2011)

2.1.4.1.2. Phase III Trial

A phase III trial reported by Herbst compared bevacizumab and erlotinib with erlotinib alone as second-line therapy for NSCLC (Herbst et al., 2011). Cases of squamous cell carcinoma were eligible if the lesion was peripheral. Treatment was given until progression or the toxic effect became unmanageable. The median overall survival times for the 317 patients treated with erlotinib alone (9.2 months) and the 319 patients treated with the combination (9.3 months) were similar. The progression-free survival time for the bevacizumab-erlotinib group (3.4 months) was significantly longer than that of the erlotinib group (1.7 months). But 130 (42%) of the 313 patients in the bevacizumab-erlotinib group had a serious adverse event, while 114 (36%) of those treated with erlotinib alone had such an event. It was concluded that the study is negative because the primary end-point of overall survival was not reached.

2.1.4.1.3. Erlotinib and Bevacizumab: Future Directions

The results of the ATLAS trial, in which two therapies with different targets were combined, may provide a further improved treatment (Miller et al., 2009). Those patients who responded to the bevacizumab-based first-line therapy with an objective response or stable disease were given bevacizumab combined with erlotinib as maintenance therapy. The trial met its primary endpoint with a significant (28%) decrease in the risk of progression and an increase in the median PFS of 1.1 months. Data on overall survival have not yet been presented and are awaited with great interest.

2.1.4.2. Sunitinib

Sunitinib (S) is a small molecule that is given orally. It inhibits several receptor tyrosine kinases, including those of platelet-derived growth factor receptors (PDGFRs), VEGFRs, stem cell factor receptor (c-KIT), Flt-3, colony-stimulating factor receptor type 1, and the glial cell line-derived neurotrophic factor receptor (RET) (Mendel et al., 2003; O'Farrell et al., 2003). It was a logical to assess the clinical efficacy of sutinib combined with bevacizumab for treating lung cancer because sunitib has a high affinity for PDGFR and Flt-3, which are implicated in angionesis but are not targeted by bevacizumab.

Table 5. Main clinical trials of bevacizumab combined with erlotinib. PFS: progression free survival. OS: overall survival

Authors	Drugs	Patients	Response rate	Toxicity
Phase II Herbst et al.,2005	Bevacizumab (15 mg/kg) + Erlotinib	n=40	PFS: 6.2 months OS: 12.6 months	1 grade 4 infection
Phase II Herbst et al., 2007	- Arm A: Bevacizumab 15 mg/kg + chemotherapy - Arm B: Bevacizumab (15 mg/kg) + Erlotinib - Arm C: chemotherapy	n=120	PFS: Arm A= 4.8 months Arm B= 4.4 months Arm C= 3 months OS: Arm A= 12.6 months Arm B= 13.7 months Arm C= 8.6 months	1 grade 5 hemorrage in arm B 2 grade 5 hemorrage in arm A
Phase II Dingemans et al., 2011	Bevacizumab 15 mg/kg+ Erlotinib	n=47	PFS : 3.8 months OS: 6.9 months No influence of KRas or EGFR mutation	0 grade 3/4 hemorrage
Phase III Herbst et al., 2011	Arm A: Bevacizumab 15 mg/kg+ Erlotinib Arm B: Erlotinib alone (2nd line)	n=636	PFS: Arm A= 3.4 months Arm B= 1.7 months OS: Arm A= 9.2 months Arm B= 9.3 months	Similar between group
Phase II Tanaka et al., 2011	Bevacizumab 15 mg/kg+ Erlotinib	n=80 (estimation)	PFS : in progress OS: in progress	

A phase I/II trial was carried out in which advanced NSCLC patients given carboplatin/paclitaxel/bevacizumab (PCB) with or without increasing doses of sunitinib (Socinski et al., 2010). Thus, 26 patients were given PCB and 30 were given PCB plus 25 mg sunitinib. Because of tolerance issues, none of the patients was given 37.5 mg suntinib. The dose of sunitinib given to 35 % of the patients on PCB plus sunitinib had to have their dose reduced, the sunitinib treatment of 52% of these patients had to be interrupted, and 59% discontinued sunitinib because of adverse, most frequently hematologic, events (neutropenia, thrombocytopenia, and leukopenia) and fatigue. The bevacizumab had to be interrupted for more patients given PCB plus sunitinib (38%) than for those on PCB alone (19%) and it had to be discontinued for more of them (52%) than for the patients on PCB alone (35%) because of adverse, mostly hematologic, events. Suprisingly, toxicity was mostly due to hematologic events. Pulmonary haemorrhage was not clearly indentified but did not seem to be the most frequently observed adverse event. The authors concluded that adding sunitinib to PCB was not well tolerated and recommended that this combination should not be studied further at these doses and schedules.

2.1.5. Clinical Trials of Bevacizumab in Elderly Patients

Patients 75 years of age or older are often excluded from clinical trials because they tend to be more fragile than younger ones. However, the recent increase in life expectancy means that older patients with an NSCLC are no longer uncommon. We have summarized the results of two phase III studies on ederly patients to determine whether bevacizumab is more toxic for elderly patients (Ramalingam et al., 2008; Leighl et al., 2010).

The ECOG 4599 study found that elderly patients, at least 70 year-old, seemed to respond better to carboplatin-paclitaxel-bevacizumab (29%) than to carboplatin paclitaxel (17%) and their progression-free survival was longer (5.9 months) on carboplatin-paclitaxel-bevacizumab than on carboplatin paclitaxel (4.9 months) (Ramalingam, JCO, 2008). The overall survival times were similar for the bevacizumab-carboplatin-paclitaxel group (11.3 months) and for the carboplatin paclitaxel group (12.1 months).

Almost all (87 %) of the elderly patients on bevacizumab plus chemotherapy suffered from grade 3 to 5 toxicities, while only 61% of those on chemotherapy alone did. Elderly patients on bevacizumab and chemotherapy were more likely to suffer from grade 3 to 5 neutropenia, bleeding, and proteinuria than younger patients. The European study (Leighl et al., 2008) also evaluated 304 elderly patients.

The progression-free survival time of the patients aged 65 years or older given bevacizumab and chemotherapy (cisplatin-gemcitabine) was longer than that for the patients given the chemotherapy with placebo, with a hazard ratio of 0.71 for the 7.5 mg/kg dosage and 0.84 for the 15 mg/kg dose. The objective response rates were 40 % for those given 7.5 mg/kg bevacizumab, 29 % for those given15 mg/kg bevacizumab, and 30% for the patients given the placebo.

The overall survival times for all three groups were similar. Frequencies of grade ≥3 toxicity were also similar for all three groups but also with younger patients. These results did not change when the cut-off used was 70 years of age. The SAiL study also analysed the responses of elderly (over 65) patients (Laskin et al., 2012). They assessed the progression-free survival time and overall survival of these older patients treated with bevacizumab and chemotherapy.

The incidences of adverse events in elderly and younger patients were similar. Any grade bleeding occurred in 38.2% of elderly patients and in 38.3% of younger patients and serious adverse events in 45.3 % of elderly patients and in 34.7% of younger patients. The median overall survival times for elderly and younger patients were similar (14.6 months) as were the times to progression (8.2 months for the elderly patients and 7.6 months for the younger patients).

A *post hoc* comparison of patients over 70 years and those younger than 70 years gave similar results. We believe that the cut-off used in these studies is probably to low because toxicity is probably greater for patients 80 older than for patients younger than 80. All these data are indirect results provided by subgroup analysis, but Spigel et al. recently conducted a phase II randomized controlled trial on 110 patients over 70 years old with advanced NSCLC to compare treatment with pemetrexed/gemcitabine/bevacizumab (cohort A) with pemetrexed/carboplatin/bevacizumab (cohort B) (Spigel et al., 2012).

Unfortunately, this study included no control arm without bevacizumab. The time to progression was 4.7 months and the overall survival time was 7.5 months for the patients in cohort A and these times were 10.2 months and 14.8 months for those in cohort B. The frequencies of grade $\geq$ 3 toxicities in the two groups were similar. Three potential treatment-related deaths occurred in cohort A (sepsis, thrombocytopenia, and myocardial infarction) and two in cohort B (sepsis and pulmonary hemorrhage). We know of no trial that has specifically compared chemotherapy plus bevacizumab to chemotherapy alone.

2.1.6. Predictive Markers

2.1.6.1. Current Concepts

Bevacizumab increases the overall survival time in both clinical trial and real life, but some patients do not response to this therapy. The greatest challenge in using bevacizumab to treat patients with NSCLC is to identify predictive biomarkers that can identify patients most likely to respond to it. Jubb et al. have explored the potential of VEGF, thrombospondin-2 and microvessel density as predictive marker for bevacizumab therapy in metastatic colorectal cancer, for which bevacizumab is also approved (Jubb et al., 2008). Their results suggest that adding bevacizumab to chemotherapy improves survival regardless the concentration of VEGF or thrombospondin-2, or the microvessel density. This trial, assessing predictive markers for the use of bevacizumab in colorectal cancer, found no marker that could identify patients who would survive longer when treated with bevacizumab. Thus, bevacizumab is used with no restriction in colo-rectal cancer.

The E4599 trial evaluated predictive markers for the use of bevacizumab to treat lung cancer (Dowlati et al., 2008). This phase II/phase III trial examined 878 patients who were given carboplatin plus paclitaxel (PC) alone or PC with bevacizumab (BPC). The survival and progression-free survival of the patienst given BPC were better than those for patients given PC. The plasma concentrations of VEGF, basic fibroblast growth factor (bFGF), soluble intercellular adhesion molecule (ICAM) and E-selectin were analysed in this cohort. The baseline ICAM concentrations were prognostic for survival and predicted the response to chemotherapy with or without bevacizumab. The VEGF concentrations prediced only the response to bevacizumab and not survival. However, bevacizumab is still given to NSCLC patients with no selection.

2.1.6.2. Future Directions

Imaging is being used to monitor predictive markers in targeted therapy. A recent trial by de Langen et al. used 18F-fluorodesoxyglucose (FDG) positon-emission tomography (PET), $H_2{}^{15}O$ PET, and dynamic contrast-enhanced magnetic resonance imaging to assess the glucose metabolism, perfusion, and microvascular permeability of lung tumor 3 weeks after bevacizumab treatment (de Langen et al., 2011). Of the 44 patients included, 40 underwent 18F-FDG PET.

The standardized glucose uptake and tumor perfusion decreased by over 20% and the progression-free survival was significantly longer (9.7 months) than in controls (2.8 months). Whole-tumor Ktrans (the endothelial transfer constant) evaluated by magnetic resonance imaging was not associated with any change in progression-free survival, but patients whose tumor Ktrans values increased by more than 15% at 3 week had shorter progression-free survival times (2.3 months) than the others (7.0 months). PET and dynamic contrast-enhanced MRI identified patients who had benefited from the bevacizumab treatment. Larger clinical trials are now needed to determine whether molecular imaging is relevant for analysing the therapeutic response to bevacizumab.

2.1.7. Anti-VEGFR2: Ramucirumab

Ramucirumab is a fully human monoclonal antibody that specifically inhibits VEGFR-2 (Spratlin et al., 2011). In vivo studies with the mouse surrogate of ramucirumab, DC101, was used to treat a mouse bearing a 54A (small cell lung carcinoma) xenograft. DC101 treatment significantly decreased the dose of radiation needed to control 50% of tumors locally (Kozin et al., 2001).

These authors also showed that adding DC101 to radiotherapy induced a delayed growth of the 54A tumor 2.2-fold compared to treatment-naive mice treated for the first time. NSCLC patients in a forthcoming phase II clinical trial will be treated with ramucirumab plus cisplatin-based doublet chemotherapy or chemotherapy alone (ImClone LLC, NCT01160744).

The primary endpoint for the 280 patients estimated to be enrolled will be progression-free survival.

The trial will close in June 2012. Another phase II clinical trial will assess the proportion of NSCLC patients treated with ramucirumab/carboplatin/paclitaxel (ImClone LLC, NCT00735696) who are progression-free at 6 months. Finally, a phase III trial on NSCLC patients previously treated will be given second line therapy consisting of ramucirumab plus docetaxel or docetaxel plus placebo. The primary endpoint will be the overall survival time (ImClone LLC, NCT01168973). This trial is still recruiting participants.

2.1.8. Fab Anti-VEGF: Ranibizumab

Ranibizumab is a monoclonal antibody fragment (Fab) derived from the same parent mouse antibody as bevacizumab. It is much smaller than the parent molecule and has been affinity matured to provide stronger binding to VEGF-A. It is approved for treating age-related macular degeneration but it has not yet been assessed for treating NSCLC (Patel et al., 2011).

2.2. Anti-HER Antibodies

2.2.1. EGFR and Signaling Pathways

The epidermal growth factor (EGFR) family of molecules was originally called the ERBB protein family because of their similarity to the erythroblastoma virus gene product, v-erbB. It is a subclass I of the receptor tyrosine kinase (RTK) superfamily and has four members: EGFR (or ERBB1), ERBB2 (or HER2), ERBB3 and ERBB4 (Hynes and Lane, 2005). All these proteins are composed of an extracellular ligand-binding region, a single membrane-spanning region and a cytoplasmic tyrosine-kinase-containing domain. The ERBB receptors are present in various tissues of epithelial, mesenchymal and neuronal origin. The binding of ligands to ERBB receptors causes them to form homo- and heterodimers and activates their intrinsic kinase domain. This results in phosphorylation of specific tyrosine residues within the cytoplasmic tail. These phosphorylated residues serve as docking sites for a range of proteins, the recruitment of which leads to activation of intracellular signaling pathways (Hynes et al., 2005). The ligands of EGFR are members of the EGF family and can be divided into three groups. The first includes EGF, transforming growth factor-α (TGF-α) and amphiregulin, which binds specifically to EGFR (ERBB1). The second includes betacellulin, heparin-binding EGF (HB-EGF) and epiregulin, which has a dual specificity, binding to both EGFR and ERBB4. The third group includes the neuregulins (NRGs), with two subgroups based on their capacity to bind to ERBB3 or ERBB4. No ligand has been clearly identified that binds to ERBB2 (HER2).

2.2.1.1. ERBB1 (EGFR)

The binding of a ligand to EGFR results in the receptor forming a homo-dimer or a heterodimer with another ERBB receptor. Several tyrosine-based motifs recruit signal transducers to the phosphorylated form of ERBB1, such as the adaptor proteins growth-factor-receptor bound-2 (GRB2) and Src-homology-2-containing (Shc), which are responsible for recruiting Ras, which activates the mitogen-activated protein kinase (MAPK) cascade containing Raf, MEK 1/2 and ERK 1/2 (Figure 2) (Nishinaka et al., 2001; Sebolt-Leopold et al., 2004; Rasul et al., 2009). Phosphorylated ERK1/2 moves to the nucleus and activates various transcription factors such as ELK1. EGFR also activates phosphatidylinositol 3-kinase (PI3K). The activated kinase phosphorylates phosphatidylinositol 4,5-biphosphate to form phosphatidylinositol 3,4,5-triphosphate, which then activates Akt (Vivanco et al., 2002). Phosphorylated Akt has several effects in the cytoplasm and in the nucleus. Phosphatidylinositol 4,5-biphosphate is hydrolyses by phospholipase c-γ (PLCγ) to diacylglycerol (DAG) and inositol triphosphate (IP3). IP3 mediates the release of calcium from intracellular stores, whereas DAG is a cofactor for the activation of the serine/threonine kinase protein kinase-C (PKC). The activation of PKC results in cell-cycle progression, transformation, differentiation and apoptosis (Oliva et al., 2005). Phosphorylation of the epidermal growth factor receptor (EGFR) can directly or indirectly activate the signal transducers and activators of transcription 1 (STAT1), STAT3 and STAT5. The activated STAT proteins move to the nucleus and directly regulate the expression of genes crucial for cell survival, proliferation, transformation and oncogenesis (Bowman et al., 2000).

EGFR is frequently present on NSCLC and tumor cells produce transforming growth factor-α (TGF-α), amphiregulin, and epidermal growth factor (EGF), which can bind to and activate cell surface EGFR (Rush et al., 1997, Carpenter et al., 1979). Overproduction of EGFR and its ligands does not seem to be associated with a poor prognosis in NSCLC, unlikely in other cancers (Rush, et al., 1997).

EGFRs control key intracellular pathways that govern fundamental cellular processes like proliferation, cell migration, metabolism, and survival. Several inhibitors of the EGFR signaling pathway have been developed; these include small molecule inhibitors of the receptor tyrosine kinase and monoclonal antibodies to the EGFR. This section focuses on the mAb.

2.2.1.2. ERBB2 (HER2)

Although ERBB2 does not interact with EGF-like ligands, it is the preferred heterodimer partner of the other three ERBB members (Tzahar et al., 1996). ERBB2 binds to a much larger subset of phosphotyrosine-binding proteins than the other ligand-binding ERBB receptors. Furthermore, ERBB2-containing heterodimers have a greater affinity and broader specificity for various ligands than the other heterodimeric receptor complexes. They probably act by prolonging the recruitment of multiple signaling pathways (Tzahar et al., 1996).

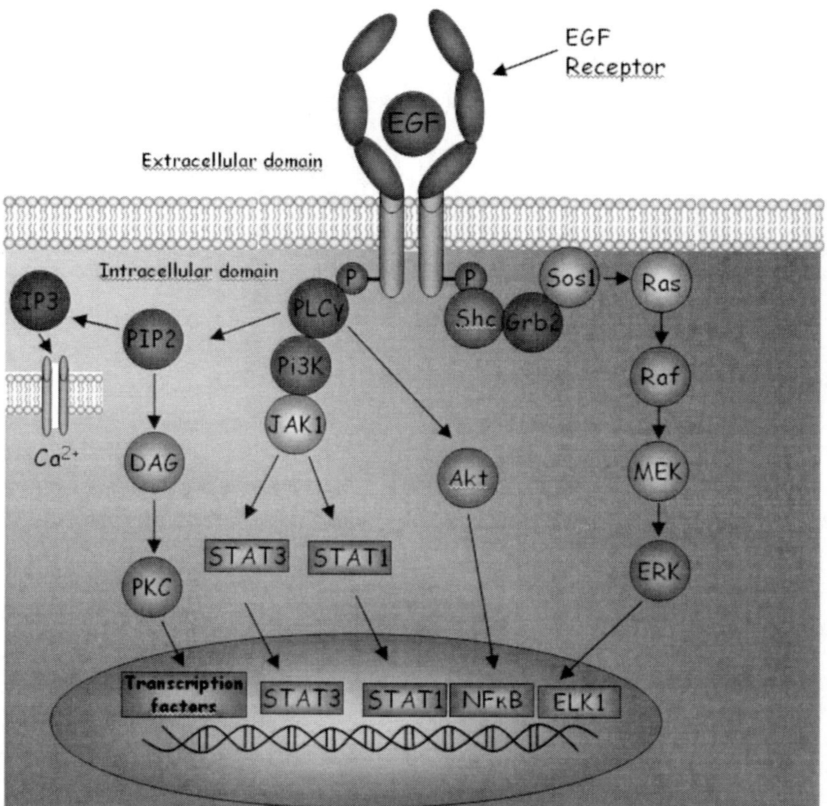

Figure 2. EGFR signalling pathway. DAG: diacylglycerol; EGF: epidermal growth factor; ERK: Extracellular signal-regulated kinases; GRB2: Growth-factor-receptor bound-2; JAK1: Janus kinase 1; Pi3k: Phosphoinositide 3-kinase; PLCγ: phospholipase Cγ; Shc: Src-homology-2-containing; STAT1: signal transducers and activators of transcription 1.

ERBB2 is infrequently overproduced in NSCLC, but it seems to be associated with a poor prognosis (Tateishi et al., 1991). HER2 was overabundant in only 20% of 563 NSCLC samples by immunohistochemistry, and in only 2% by FISH (Heinmoller et al., 2003). Another study found that HER2 was overabundant in 20% of samples by a combination immunochemistry and FISH (Tan et al., 2003). Patients whose NSCLC reacts positively for HER-2/neu protein tended to have shorter survival times.

Yet another study on 102 NSCLC patients evaluated the number of copies of the HER2 gene per cell by FISH and the HER2 protein immunohistochemically (Cappuzo et al., 2005). It found that 22.8% of patients had high number of copies of the HER2 gene but that only 7% of them were immunochemically positive for HER2.

2.2.2. Cetuximab: Anti-EGFR Antibody

2.2.2.1. Pre-Clinical Studies

Raben et al. assessed the amounts of EGFR in different NSCLC or SCLC cell lines and found that it was more abundant in H292 cells (lung mucoepidermoid carcinoma) than in H332 cells (small cell lung cancer cell line), A549 (lung adenocarcinoma), H157 (squamous cell carcinoma), and Calu3 cells (lung adenocarcioma) (Raben et al., 2005). It's concentration was very low in H358 cells (bronchioloalveolar carcinoma). The only line that had no EGFR was H520 (squamous cell carcinoma). *In vivo,* cetuximab significantly inhibited the growth of H292 and H332, the cell lines with most EGFR, and Calu-3, with an intermediate EGFR content, whereas it was less efficient at inhibiting A549 and H358 cels and did not inhibit the growth of H157 cells, whose EGFR content is similar to that of A549 (Raben et al., 2005). These results suggest that cetuximab activity is not correlated with the abundance of EGFR in NSCLC.

Cetuximab (3-100 nmol/L) and radiation (2-6 Gy) acted strongly in synergy to inhibit the growth of the cetuximab-sensitive cell lines H292, and H322, and also that of the less responsive lines A549, Calu-3 and H358. Similarly, the response of these cell lines to cisplatin plus cetuximab was greater than the response to cetuximab alone (Raben et al., 2005). Cetuximab plus radiation decreased volume of xenografted H292 tumors with significantly more than cetuximab alone or radiation alone or the control (Raben et al., 2005). Another study found that chemotherapy (cisplatin, gemcitabine or docetaxel) plus cetuximab had a greater antitumor effect on H292 xenografts than chemoptherapy or cetuximab alone (Steinert et al., 2007).

2.2.2.2. Preclinical Studies on the Pulmonary Administered of Cetuximab

Blood is the conventional delivery route for antibody-based therapeutics. However, some small studies have reported relative partioning to the lung from serum, with only a low concentration of antibody-based therapeutics reaching the lungs (Hart et al, 2001, Dall'Acqua et al 2006; Vugmeyster et al., 2010). When examining the dosing route to deliver mAbs into the lungs, the airways offer several potential advantages over systemic and oral routes, including loco-regional delivery to the lungs providing high drug concentration, avoidance of the first-pass metabolic degradation in the liver and reduction of systemic side effects. The pulmonary route is the accepted standard route for key respiratory drugs for COPD and asthma including b2-adrenoceptor agonists, muscarinic antagonists, and corticosteroids -

mainly to maintain an acceptable therapeutic index. At the present time, with the exception of Pulmozyme® a Rh-DNase used in cystic fibrosis, the airways is mainly used with small molecule drugs such as corticoids and antibiotics. A few years ago we began to investigate the local, pulmonary, delivery of mAbs to determine whether this route improved pharmacokinetics and therapeutic efficacy of mAbs while limiting their systemic toxicity. We first determined whether mAb resisted the aerosolization process. We found that mAbs are sensitive to aerosolization. Their molecular structure is altered by nebulization with certain types of devices so that they form aggregates that are potentially immunogenic and the pharmacology of the mAb is altered. We tested three technologies and found that the mesh nebulizer seemed to have the least effect on cetuximab, cetuximab remained immunologically intact and its pharmacological properties unchanged, as assessed by *in vitro* assays. In addition, few if any aggregates were formed and the sizes of the aerosol particles generated were well suited for pulmonary deposition within the respiratory zone (Maillet et al., 2008).

We evaluated the pharmacokinetics and distribution of aerosolized cetuximab in a xenogeneic model of A431 intrabronchially engrafted in nude mice (Maillet et al, 2011). We conjugated the cetuximab to a fluorochrome so as to follow its distribution *in vivo* by near-infrared fluorescence (NIRF) imaging for 72 hours. Imaging showed that cetuximab delivered via the airways accumulated durably in the lungs and the tumor, although the fluorescence signal observed in the liver 1 hour after delivery indicated that some mAb reached the systemic circulation. The concentrations of cetuximab in the systemic circulation were lower after pulmonary administration than after intravenous injection. The area under the concentration/time curves (AUC) estimated by the compartmental model was 73 μg.h/mL after aerosol delivery and 654 μg.h/mL after i.v. injection. The mean absorption time (MAT) was 34 h and a peak plasma concentration (Tmax) was reached at approximately 48 h. Pharmacokinetic analysis also showed that the mean absorption by the blood of airways-delivered cetuximab was low, around 11%. FcRn also seems to be implicated in the passage of IgG from the alveolar compartment into the bloodstream, as suggested by others (Bitonti et al., 2004, 2006; Dumont et al., 2005). It is difficult to extrapolate from our results to human for several reasons. First, the distributions of FcRn in rodents and humans are different. Second, cetuximab does not cross-react with murine EGFR, which probably modified its clearance. Finally, our results were obtained in immunodeficient nude mice.

We are, therefore, performing pharmacokinetic analyses in cynomolgus macaques. Our preliminary results are similar to those obtained in mice. We are also comparing the activities of aerosolized cetuximab and i.p. cetuximab in an orthotopic xenograft model to determine whether this route could be an alternative to intravenous injection.

2.2.2.3. Pharmacokinetic

The pharmacokinetic profiles of single intravenous infusions of 7.5, 24 or 75 mg/kg ofcetuximab in cynomolgus monkeys showed dose-related increases in C_{max} and AUC, dose-related decreases in clearance with an increase in apparent half-life (terminal half-life was 3 days with the lowest dose and 7 days with high dose), and a distribution volume at steady state that was approximately equal to the vascular space (data of approval file). Repeated administration of the same doses twice weekly confirmed that exposure to cetuximab was continuous over the duration of the study. Only one monkey developed anti-cetuximab antibodies in preclinical studies, with decreases in serum cetuximab concentrations.

A single dose of cetuximab serum concentration reached a maximum 1 to 2 hours after the end of infusion in humans (Humblet et al., 2004). Cetuximab is probably mainly eliminated by binding to the EGFR followed by intracellular internalisation and subsequent degradation.

The maximum observed concentration (Cmax) and the area under the curve (AUC) were proportional to the dose of cetuximab (20 to 400 mg/m2). The maximum concentrations ranged from 19.9 μg/ml with 50 mg/m2 to 243.2 μg/ml with 500 mg/mg2 (Tan et al., 2006). Clearance decreased and half-life was prolonged with increasing doses of cetuximab reaching a plateau at doses ≥ 200 mg/m^2 and a half-life of 3-4 days. The non linearity of the half-life and clearance with dose may be due to an additional saturable pathway that helps eliminate cetuximab at low doses, which is not detectable when a high initial dose of cetuximab (400 mg/m^2) is administered intravenously followed by weekly doses of 250 mg/m^2.

Thus the pharmacokinetics of cetuximab do not change with repeated administration or when combined with chemotherapy. Anti-cetuximab antibodies were uncommon (Tan et al., 2006).

The choice of dose was explained in the approval file (Merck: Data on file, Merck KGaA). Early studies on doses between 5 and 500 mg/m^2 found that the profile was acceptable up to and including 400 mg/m^2 per week. Higher doses (500 mg/m^2) resulted in unacceptable skin toxicity A pharmacodynamic analysis of the effect of cetuximab on EGFR protein showed that EGFR synthesis was maximally inhibited at doses of 250-500 mg/m^2. A dose of 250 mg/m^2 produced an increase in EGFR protein syntesis, suggesting that therapeutic activity would be best with a dose of 250 mg/m^2 of more. Several studies have found that an initial dose of 400 mg/m^2 followed by a weekly dose of 250 mg/m^2 is well tolerated and efficacious.

2.2.2.4. Clinical Trials of Cetuximab Combined with Chemotherapy

2.2.2.4.1. Phase I/II

2.2.2.4.1.1. First Line Therapy

Phase I/II trials on cetuximab combined with various chemotherapy regimens for NSCLC found significant toxicity, with skin rash and neutropenia in almost all trials. These trials were not constructed to evaluate efficiency and found a low anticancer effect. The first clinical trial of cetuximab in NSCLC was conducted by Baselga et al (Baselga et al., 2000). The 52 patients with solid tumors, including a few with lung cancer, were given cetuximab as a single dose, weekly multiple doses, or weekly multiple doses plus cisplatin. Patients given multiple doses were up to 400 mg/m^2. The pharmacokinetics, safety and response data showed that the pharmacokinetics of cetuximab were nonlinear, with antibody doses of 200 to 400 mg/m^2 being associated with complete saturation of systemic clearance. Cetuximab clearance did not change with repeated doses or when given with cisplatin. One patient given a low dose developed anti-cetuximab antibodies and his/her response was not evaluable. Toxicity was low with only 4 (8%) patients with toxicity grade ≥ 3. The most adverse event was skin toxicity with an acne-like rash. This study was not constructed to assess the clinical response, but 11 (58%) of the 19 patients whose response could be assessed at 4 weeks had stable disease, including a partial response in head and neck cancer patients. The great interest in targeted therapy has led to many phase I/II clinical trial of cetuximab combined with chemotherapy, specifically in NSCLC.

Cisplatin and-gemcitabine. The first study that specifically assessed cetuximab in NSCLC was done on 35 patients with advanced untreated NSCLC and immunohistochemical evidence of EGFR. They were given cetuximab combined with cisplatin and gemcitabine (Robert et al., 2005). An initial dose of 400 mg/m^2 was followed by weekly doses of 250 mg/m^2. The most frequently reported adverse events of cetuximab were an acne-like rash (88.6%), dry skin (34.3%), asthenia and skin disorders (31.4%), but most were mild to moderate. One patient withdrew from the study because of grade 3 allergic reactions. Myelosuppression, the most frequently observed toxicity, was linked to the chemotherapy. There were 10 partial responses (28.6%) and 21 (60 %) patients had a stable disease. The median time to progression was 5.5 months, and the median overall survival was 10 months.

A study to compare cetuximab combined with chemotherapy with chemotherapy alone as first line therapy in chemonaive NSCLC was done by Butts et al. on 131 patients (Butts et al., 2007). They were given cetuximab combined with cisplatin or carboplatin and gemcitabine (arm A), or chemotherapy alone (arm B). In arm A, 18 patients (27.7%) had partial responses, as did 12 (18.2%) in arm B. The median progression-free survival time was 5.09 months for arm A and 4.21 months in arm B. The median overall survival time was 11.99 months in arm A and 9.26 months in arm B. Skin rash toxicity was observed in 73% of patients in arm A and 11 % of the patients in arm B. Severe infusion reactions related to treatment occurred in three patients given cetuximab, whereas none occurred in patients on chemotherapy alone. Hematological adverse events in the two groups were similar. These data suggest that adding cetuximab to chemotherapy improves clinical outcomes.

Carboplatin or cisplatin and paclitaxel. Preclinical studies showed that paclitaxel and cetuximab acted in synergy to inhibit tumor growth in a murine orthotopic bladder carcinoma model (Inoue et al., 2000). Therefore cetuximab combined with cisplatin/paclitaxel was assessed in clinical trials. The first trial was on 31 patients with untreated metastatic NSCLC who were given cetuximab combined with carboplatin/paclitaxel, the reference treatment as first line therapy for NSCLC in the USA. The most common cetuximab toxicity was a rash in 84% of patients (grade 3 in 13%). Grade 3 toxicities were rare, with 4% of patients developing grade 3 neutropenia or thrombocytopenia. There was no allergic reaction. Pharmacokinetic sampling showed no interaction between carboplatin, paclitaxel, and cetuximab. An objective response was observed in eight patients (26%). The median time to progression was 5 months and the median survival time was 11 months. A single arm study on 53 NSCLC patients tested cetuximab plus carboplatin/paclitaxel (Borghaei et al., 2008). Paclitaxel was given weekly and carboplatin every month. Cetuximab was delivered weekly and continued weekly until progression or toxicity became unmanageable. The response rate was 57%, with 3 complete responses and 27 partial responses. The estimated overall survival time was 13.8 months with an event-free survival time of 5.53 months. Women survived longer than men, and survival was improved if there had been no prior radiation, if general status was good and immunohistochemistry showed the presence of epidermal growth factor receptors. Toxicities included a rash (28% grade 3), nail changes (3.7% grade 3) and neutropenia (25% grade 3 and 13% grade 4). The two-arm phase II study of Socinsky et al. compared the effects of two schedules of paclitaxel/carboplatin plus weekly cetuximab on 168 advanced or metastatic NSCLC patients (Socinsky et al., 2009). EGFR status was not assessed. Patients in arm A were given cetuximab plus paclitaxel (225 mg/m^2)/carboplatin (AUC6) every 3 weeks, while those in arm B were given cetuximab plus paclitaxel (100 mg/m^2) on days 1, 8, and 15 every 3 weeks and carboplatin (AUC6) on day 1 and every 4 weeks. A maximum of four cycles was administered and patients with a complete response, partial response, or stable disease after four cycles were given cetuximab weekly until disease progression or toxicity became unacceptable. The median progression-free survival time, defined as the primary endpoint, was 4.7 months for arm A and 4.3 months for arm B (6-month PFS for arm A: 27.3% and 30.9% for arm B). The median overall survival time was 11.4 for arm A and 9.8 months for arm B. The objective response rate was 29.6% for arm A and 25% for arm B. There was no difference between the two schedules but grade 4 neutropenia was more frequent in arm B (18.5%) than in arm A (3.6%). A trial to determine the best regimen to use in a phase III trial was carried out on 224 chemotherapy-naive patients with advanced-stage NSCLC. One arm (A) was given paclitaxel (225 mg/m^2) and carboplatin (area under the curve, 6) every 3 weeks plus concurrent cetuximab (400 mg/m^2 initial dose followed by 250 mg/m^2 weekly) for four cycles followed by maintenance cetuximab. The other was given sequential paclitaxel-carboplatin for four cycles followed by cetuximab (Herbst et al., 2010). The median overall survival time was 10.9 months for patients receiving concurrent therapy (arm A) and 10.7 months for patientsgiven sequential therapy (arm B). The response rates and progression-free survival times in the two arms were similar (32% and 4.3 months for arm A and 30 % and 4.4 months for arm B). Toxicity in the two groups was also similar, excluding sensory neuropathy, which was significantly higher in arm A (15%) than in arm B (5%). Although the two regimens met the efficacy criterion for continued evaluation, the concurrent paclitaxel/carboplatin plus cetuximab regimen was chosen for phase III study.

Carboplatin and docetaxel. The 80 chemonaïve NSCLC patients in a single-arm phase II trial were given cetuximab combined with carboplatin and docetaxel for up to 6 cycles. Maintenance cetuximab was then given alone for 1 year or until disease progression (Belani et al., 2008). The objective response rate, the primary endpoint, was 15.2% (1 patient had a complete response and 11 had partial responses). The median progression-free survival time was 4.6 months and 4 patients (14%) remained free of disease progression at 12 months. The median overall survival time was 10.3 months. The main grade ≥3 adverse event was neutropenia (30%). The authors concluded that this combination had a small anticancer effect.

Cisplatin and vinorelbine. The 86 NSCLC patients with EGFR overproduction who took part in a two-arm phase II trial were given cisplatin on day 1 and vinorelbine on days 1 and 8 every 3 weeks for up to 8 cycles (arm A) or these chemotherapy drugs combined with weekly cetuximab (arm B) (Rosell et al., 2008). The arm B patients were allowed to continue cetuximab until desease progression or toxicity became unmanageable. Confirmed response rates were 28% in arm A and 35% in arm B. The median progression-free survival time was 4.6 months in arm A and 5.0 months in arm B, with PFS rates at 12 months of 0% in arm A and 15% in arm B. The median overall survival time was 7.3 months in arm A and 8.3 months in arm B. The 24-month survival rates were 0% in arm Aand 16% in arm B. The cetuximab combination was well tolerated. The grade ≥3 adverse events, which occurred mostly in arm B, were skin rash and neutropenia. These preliminary data suggest that the skin rash was correlated with the response rate.

Gemcitabine. The combination of gemcitabine with cetuximab was assessed in elderly patients (older than 70 years) with stage IV or IIIB NSCLC and adults younger than 70 years with a poor general status (Gridelli et al., 2010). One group of patients was given concomitant treatment (gemcitabine, for a maximum of 6 cycles, plus cetuximab until progression) (arm A) and the other sequential treatment (gemcitabine, for a maximum of 6 cycles, followed by cetuximab) (arm B). In arm B, 34.5% of the elderly patients and 60.0% of the patients with poor performance status could not be given cetuximab after gemcitabine. The 1-year survival rates for the elderly patients were 41.4% for arm A and 31.0% for arm B and for the poor performance status adult patients they were 27.3% for arm A and 35.0% for arm B. Toxicity in the two treatment groups was similar, but allergic response occurred only in the elderly patients. The elderly patients in arm A, but not the others, who developed skin toxicity within the first two cycles of treatment survived longer. Sequential treatment cannot be proposed for further trials because of poor compliance and inconsistent survival outcomes.

Docetaxel-Gemcitabine. Cetuximab combined with an uncommon regimen (docetaxel and gemcitabine) was also assessed in 69 NSCLC patients who had not been treated (Spigel et al., 2010). The primary endpoint, an overall response rate $\geq$ 25%, was not reached because only 17% had an objective response.

The median progression-free time was 4 months and the overall survival time was 9.4 months. The most common grade $\geq$ 3 toxicities were neutropenia (25%), rash (22%), and fatigue (12%). The trial was stopped because of a higher-than-anticipated rate of cetuximab-related severe hypersensitivity reactions in 4 patients of the first 12 enrolled, including 1 fatal event. This regimen was severely toxic and thus should not be repeated.

2.2.2.4.1.2. Second Line Therapy

Cetuximab alone. A group of 66 NSCLC patients with recurrent or progressive NSCLC who had been treated with at least one chemotherapy regimen were given cetuximab weekly in a phase II trial (Hanna et al., 2008). EGFR expression was indifferent. The primary endpoint was the response rate and the secondary endpoints were an estimation of time to progression and survival time (Table 7). Grade 3/4 toxicities included acne-like rash (6.1%), anaphylactic reactions (1.5%), and diarrhea (1.5%). The response rate for all patients was only 4.5% and the stable disease rate was 30.3%. The response rate for patients with EGFR-positive tumors (n = 60) was 5%. The median time to progression for all patients was 2.3 months and the median survival time was 8.9 months.

Docetaxel. This phase II trial determined the response rate, survival, safety, and pharmacokinetics (PK) of cetuximab combined with docetaxel as a second line therapy for chemotherapy-refractory/resistant patients with advanced NSCLC and overexpression of EGFR (Kim et al., 2008).

The confirmed responses included 1 complete response (1.8%), 10 partial responses (18.2%), and 20 with stable disease (36.4%). The response rate was 20% and the median time to disease progression was 3.5 months. The median overall survival (OS) time was 7.5 months with a 1-year survival rate of 35%. There were no differences in PK parameters of docetaxel alone or with cetuximab. The most common grade $\geq$ 3 adverse events were leukopenia (27.3%) and skin rash (21.8%). Four patients (7.3%) discontinued due to allergic reactions, but no details were given.

Table 6. Main clinical trials of cetuximab alone or combined with chemotherapy as first line therapy in NSCLC. Cetuximab was given with an initial dose of 400 mg/m^2 followed by weekly dose of 250 mg/m^2 except for trial conducted by Baselga et al. PC: Paclitaxel/Carboplatin; D/Gem: Carboplatin/Gemcitabine. Pem. Pemetrexed. Cis/Gem: Cisplatin/Gemcitabine; Cis/Vin: cisplatin/vinorelbin. CD: carboplatin/docetaxel; PFS: progression free survival; OS: overall survival

Authors	Drugs	Patients	Response rate	Toxicity
Phase I Baselga et al., 2000	Cetuximab 200 to 400 mg/m^2 in various cancer	n=52	No response in NSCLC patients	acne-like rash
Phase II Robert et al., 2005	Cetuximab + Cis/Gem	n=35	PFS : 5.5 months OS: 10 months	Acne-like rash (88.6%), Dry skin (34.3%), Skin disorders (31.4%)
Phase II Butts et al., 2007	Arm A: Cetuximab + Cis/Gem Arm B: Cis/Gem alone	n=131	PFS: Arm A= 5.09 months Arm B= 4.21 months OS: Arm A= 11.99 months Arm B= 9.26 months	Arm A: Skin rash (78%) Severe infusion reaction in 3 patients Arm B: Skin rash (11%)
Phase II Inoue et al., 2000	Cetuximab + PC	n=31	PFS : 5 months OS: 11 months	Rash: 84% Grade ≥3 rash : 13%
Phase II Borghaei et al., 2008	Cetuximab+ PC	n=53	PFS : 5.53 months OS: 13.8 months	Grade ≥3 rash : 28% Grade ≥3 neutropenia: 25%
Phase II Socinsky et al., 2009	Arm A: Cetuximab + PC every 3 weeks Arm B : Cetuximab + PC with P weekly	n=168	PFS: Arm A= 4.7 months Arm B= 4.3 months OS: Arm A= 11.4 months Arm B= 9.8 months	Arm A: grade 4 neutropenia (18.5%) Arm B: grade 4 neutropenia (3.6%)
Phase II Herbst et al., 2010	Arm A cetuximab + concurrent PC Arm B: cetuximab + sequential PC	n=224	PFS: Arm A= 4.3 months Arm B= 4.4 months OS: Arm A= 10.9 months Arm B= 10.7 months	
Phase II Betani et al., 2008	Cetuximab+ CD	n=80	PFS: 4.6 months OS: 10.6 months	Grade ≥3 neutropenia: 30%
Phase II Rosell et al., 2008	Arm A : Cis/Vin alone Arm B : cetuximab + Cis/Vin	n=86	PFS: Arm A= 4.6 months Arm B= 5.0 months OS: Arm A= 7.3 months Arm B= 8.3 months	
Phase II Gridelly et al., 2010	Arm A concomitant cetuximab/Gem Arm B: Gem followed by cetuximab	n=100 Elderly or poor general status	- Elderly patients PFS: Arm A= 2.9 months Arm B= 3.8 months OS: Arm A= 5.7 months Arm B= 8.6 months - Adults patients with poor general status PFS: Arm A= 5.5 months Arm B= 2.1 months OS: Arm A= 9.5 months Arm B= 6.2 months	
Phase II Spigel et al., 2010	Cetuximab + D/Gem	n=69	PFS: 4 months OS: 9.4 months	Stopped because of high severe hypersensitivity reaction

Pemetrexed. A few years ago there was great interest in pemetrexed for treating NSCLC and it is now approved for non-squamous NSCLC. This phase I/II trial examined a combination of cetuximab and pemetrexed in 36 NSCLC patients with recurrent NSCLC (any histology) (Jalal et al., 2009). All the patients had previously been given at least one platinum-based chemotherapy regimen. They were given cetuximab weekly with increasing doses of pemetrexed every 3 weeks in a phase I portion. Once the maximum tolerated dose of the combination was determined, patients were enrolled in the phase II trial portion with the median time to disease progression as the primary endpoint. The median time to progression was 3.5 months. The median survival time was 10 months and the 1-year survival rate was 38.5%. The clinical benefit rate (defined as complete responses, partial responses and stable diseases) was 69.2%. The most common toxicities were acne-like rash, fatigue, mucositis, and nausea, but there were no allergic reactions. The authors concluded that the combined regimen did not seem to improve the time to disease progression over historical controls of any single agent. However, this study was too small and underpowered to be conclusive.

2.2.2.4.1.3. Bronchioloalveolar Carcinoma

Bronchioloalveolar carcinoma (BAC) is a subtype of NSCLC with distinct pathological features and clinical behavior. It accounts for approximately 5% of all cases of NSCLC. By definition, the growth pattern of BAC is lepidic with no evidence of stromal, vascular, or pleural invasion. Cetuximab therapy was assessed in 68 patients with advanced-stage pure BAC or adenocarcinoma with BAC features in the phase II trial (Ramalingam et al., 2011). Patients were included who had had up to one prior chemotherapy regimen. Cetuximab was given as a weekly intravenous infusion until disease progression or toxicity became unacceptable. Skin rash was the most common toxicity and the most severe (grade 3, 15%). The primary endpoint was not reached because the confirmed response rate was less than 50 % (7%). The disease of 35% of patients was stable. The median survival time was 13 months and the progression-free survival time was and 3.3 months. Mutation of EGFR and KRas were not correlated with the response rate. The authors found a favorable correlation between the severity of skin rash and the efficacy of cetuximab, though it was not statistically significant. They concluded that the response rate was low, with modest PFS and OS, but the results are similar to those obtained with chemotherapy.

Table 7. Main clinical trials of cetuximab alone or combined with chemotherapy as second line therapy in NSCLC. Cetuximab was given with an initial dose of 400 mg/m^2 followed by weekly dose of 250 mg/. BAC: Bronchioloalveolar carcinoma. PFS: progression free survival; OS: overall survival

Authors	Drugs	Patients	Response rate	Toxicity
Phase II Hanna et al., 2008	Cetuximab alone	n=66	PFS : 2.3 months OS: 8.9 months	acne-like rash (6.1%) anaphylactic reactions (1.5%)
Phase II Kim et al., 2008	Cetuximab + docetaxel	n=47	PFS : 3.5 months OS: 7.5 months	Grade ≥ 3 leukopenia (27.3%) and skin rash (21.8%)
Phase II Jalal et al., 2009	Cetuximab + pemetrexed	n=36	PFS: 3.5 months OS: 10 months	
Phase II Ramalingam et al., 2011	Cetuximab alone in BAC	n=	PFS : 3.3 months OS: 13 months	15 % Grade ≥ 3 skin rash

2.2.2.4.2. Phase III

The two-arm FLEX phase III trial of Pirker et al. was conducted on 1125 chemo-naïve patients with advanced NSCLC treated with cetuximab plus cisplatin and vinorelbine, or cisplatin/vinorelbine alone. Eligibility criteria included immunohistochemical evidence of EGFR expression (Pirker at al., 2009). Cetuximab was continued after the end of chemotherapy until disease progression or toxicity became unacceptable. The median overall survival time of the chemotherapy-plus-cetuximab group was significantly longer (11.3 months) than that of the chemotherapy-alone group (10.1 months) (Table 8). It is difficult to interpret these results because no data are provided about second line therapy and we know that the overall survival time is influenced by the treatment given after the first-line therapy. The progression-free survival time mainly reflects the efficacy of the first line therapy. However, The PFS of the two groups were not statistically different (4.8 months), in this trial. The toxicity profiles of the two groups were similar.

Table 8. Phase III clinical trials of cetuximab alone or combined with chemotherapy as first line therapy in NSCLC. Cetuximab was given with an initial dose of 400 mg/m^2 followed by weekly dose of 250 mg/m^2. Cis/Vin: cisplatin/vinorelbin; CT: carboplatin/taxane (paclitaxel or docetaxel). PFS: progression free survival; OS: overall survival

Authors	Drugs	Patients	Response rate	Toxicity
Phase III Pirker at al., 2009	Arm A : Cis/Vin alone Arm B : cetuximab + Cis/Vin	n=1125	PFS: Arm A= 4.8 months Arm B= 4.8 months (p=0.39) OS: Arm A=10.1 months Arm B=11.3 months(p=0.044)	Grade ≥ 3 febrile neutropenia was more frequent in the cetuximab arm (22%)
Phase II Lynch et al., 2010	Arm A Cetuximab + CT Arm B: CT alone	n=676	PFS: Arm A= 4.4 months Arm B=4.24 months OS: Arm A=9.69 months Arm B=8.38 months	

Grade ≥ 3 febrile neutropenia was statistically more frequent in the cetuximab plus cisplatin/vinorelbin group (22%) than in the chemotherapy alone group (15%). Skin rash, the most common adverse event of cetuximab, was, unsurprisingly, more frequent with cetuximab (10%) than in the chemotherapy alone group (<1%). A second phase III trial (BMS099) included 676 chemo-naïve NSCLC patients who were treated with cetuximab plus carboplatin/taxane (paclitaxel or docetaxel), or carboplatin/taxane alone (Lynch et al., 2010). As in previous trial, the progression-free survival time, the primary endpoint, was not statistically improved. The median PFS time was 4.4 months with cetuximab plus chemotherapy and 4.24 months with chemotherapy alone. The median overall survival times were also not statistically different (9.69 months with cetuximab plus chemotherapy and 8.38 months with chemotherapy alone). The overall response rate, a subjective criterion, was 25.7% with cetuximab/chemotherapy and 17.2% with chemoptherapy alone. The toxicity profiles were similar to those in the FLEX trial. Based on these two trials, cetuximab was not approved by the EMEA or the FDA. EMEA considered that the drug has no convincing effect while the toxicity was considerable.

2.2.2.4.3. Cetuximab and Other Targeted Therapies

2.2.2.4.3.1. Anti-EGFR Tyrosine Kinase Inhibitor

The rationale of combining an anti-EGFR monoclonal antibody and a tyrosine kinase inhibitor (TKI) is that blocking the different target sites on EGFR (extracellular and intracellular domains) may enhance the inhibition of downstream signaling and lead to better treatment responses and outcomes. The combination of cetuximab plus gefitinib or erlotinib enhanced the inhibition of cell growth *in vitro* more than any agent alone (Huang et al., 2004). And only the highest doses of single-agent gefitinib or cetuximab delivered alone resulted in transient complete tumor remission in a xenograft murine model of lung cancer. In contrast, suboptimal doses of gefitinib plus cetuximab resulted in the complete and permanent regression of large tumors (Matar et al., 2004). Hence, a combination of cetuximab and anti-EGFR TKI was assessed in clinical trials.

Main clinical trials combining cetuximab with targeted therapies are summarized in Table 9. Guarino et al. conducted a phase I study on 22 patients, including 14 with NSCLC, in which patients were given escalating doses of cetuximab and erlotinib to determine the optimal doses of this combination (Guarino et al., 2009). All the patients suffered from the most adverse event, a skin rash, but it was grade ≥ 3 in only 9%. The recommended doses for phase II studies were 250 mg/m^2 i.v. weekly for cetuximab and 150 mg daily orally for erlotinib. Another study concluded that the recommended doses for phase II study were 250 mg/m^2 weekly intravenous for cetuximab and 250 mg daily orally for gefitinib (Ramanligam et al., 2008).

Neal et al. evaluated the efficacy of cetuximab in 18 NSCLC patients who had disease progression despite being given an oral tyrosine kinase inhibitor (Neal et al., 2010). The average number of prior treatments was high (= 4.2). The response rate was 0/18 (0%), and 28% of patients had confirmed stable disease. The median progression-free survival time was 1.8 months and the median overall survival time was 7.5 months. Common toxicities were mild and included fatigue, skin rash, and nausea/vomiting. Two patients developed interstitial lung diseases, which was life threatening in one case.

Future directions. A clinical trial is currently in progress to assesse the efficacy of cetuximab for treating NSCLC patients who have become resistant to erlotinib as a first line therapy (Bristol-Myers Squibb, NCT00716456).

2.2.2.4.3.2. Bortezomib

Bortezomib is the first of a new class of targeted drugs that are proteasome inhibitors. Bortezomib inhibits the orderly degradation of cellular proteins by the ubiquitin–proteasome pathway, leading to the inactivation of the anti-apoptotic transcriptional regulator, nuclear factor-kB (NF-kB) (Rajkumar et al, 2005). The combination of bortezomib and cetuximab had a significant synergistic inhibitory effect on the growth of A549 lung adenocarcinoma cells (Cascone et al., 2008). The antiproliferative activity of bortezomib epidermoid carcinoma A431 cells was significantly enhanced by adding cetuximab (Wagenblast et al., 2009). Cetuximab and bortezomib were given to 37 patients with solid tumors that were immunohistochemically positive for EGFR in a phase I study to determine the maximum tolerated dose (Dudek et al., 2009). All the patients had disease progression despite at least one prior treatment and were given escalating doses of cetuximab and bortezomib. The highest dose of bortezomib tested (2.0 mg/m^2) was below the maximum tolerated dose. The outcomes included disease progression in 21 patients (56.7%) and stable disease (SD) at 6 weeks in 16 patients (43.3%). A phase II study compared a combination of docetaxel and cetuximab (armA) with docetaxel and bortezomib (arm B) as first line therapy in 59 NSCLC patients with performance status 2 (altered general status) (Lilenbaum et al., 2009). The complete or partial response rate was 13.3% in arm A and 10.3% in arm B.

The median progression-free survival time, the primary endpoint was 3.4 months in arm A and 1.9 months in arm B. Grade 3/4 hematological toxicity was 16% in arm A and 21% in arm B, whereas 63% of patients in arm A suffered nonhematological toxicities, as did 44% of patients in arm B.

Table 9. Main NSCLC clinical trials of cetuximab combined with targeted therapy. PFS: progression free survival; OS: overall survival

Authors	Drugs	Patients	Response rate	Toxicity
Phase I Guarino et al., 2009	Cetuximab + erlotinib	n=36 including 14 NSCLC	No objective response	Skin rash (100%) (Grade ≥ 3: 9%)
Phase II Ramanligam et al., 2008	Cetuximab + erlotinib	n=13	No objective response	1 case of grade 3 skin rash
Phase II Neal et al., 2010	Cetuximab in patients with progression under erlotinib	n=18	No objective response PFS: 1.8 months OS: 7.5 months	
Phase I Dudek et al., 2009	Cetuximab + bortezomib	n=37	No objective response	Grade ≥ 3 fatigue (22%), dyspnoea (16%), infection (11%)
Phase II Lilenbaum et al., 2009	Arm A: Cetuximab + docetaxel Arm B: Bortezomib + docetaxel	n=59	PFS: Arm A= 3.4 months Arm B= 1.9 months OS: Arm A= 5 months Arm B= 3.9 months	Grade ≥ 3 nonhematological toxicity: Arm A= 63% Arm B= 44%

The combination of docetaxel and cetuximab seemed to be superior but the primary endpoint was not reached. This combination should not be used for further investigation. No phase III study has yet started.

2.2.2.4.4. Cetuximab and radiotherapy

The combination modality chemotherapy and radiotherapy conferred a small but significant survival advantage over radiotherapy alone (Alberti et al., 1995). Moreover, concomitant cetuximab and radiotherapy increased the local control and prolonged the survival of patients with locally advanced squamous cell carcinoma of the head and neck better than radiotherapy alone (Bonner et al., 2006). The median progression-free survival time of head and neck cancer patients treated in this trial with radiotherapy plus cetuximab was 17.1 months and 12.4 months for those treated with radiotherapy alone.

A preclinical study found that cetuximab plus radiation inhibit the growth of H292 (mucoepidermoid pulmonary carcinoma) and H322 (bronchioloalveolar carcinoma) cells much better than either agent alone (Raben et al., 2005). A combination of cetuximab plus radiation inhibited tumor growth in a murine xenograft model with H292 more than either therapy alone.

The safety of combining cetuximab and radiation was assessed in a clinical trial on 12 patients with locally advanced NSCLC (Table 10) (Hughes et al., 2008). They were given platinum-based induction chemotherapy followed by weekly intravenous cetuximab and concomitant radiotherapy (64 Gy/32 fractions/45 days). Most (9/12) patients completed the concomitant therapy as planned, with no dose reductions. Toxicity was acceptable; one patient developed a grade 2 skin reaction following the third dose of cetuximab and one patient had a grade 3 pneumonitis. The safety of cetuximab plus radiotherapy was also evaluated on 57 elderly (70 years +) patients with locally advanced NSCLC (Jatoi et al., 2010).

They were treated with cetuximab and radiotherapy as first-line therapy. Forty (70%) patients lived for more than 11 months, which exceeded the anticipated survival rate of 50%. The median survival time was 15.1 months and the median progression-free survival time was 7.2 months. No treatment-related deaths occurred. About half (31) experienced grade ≥ 3 adverse events, most commonly fatigue, anorexia, breathless, and rash, each of which occurred in <10% of patients.

A combination of cetuximab and radiotherapy (68 Gy/35 fractions/49 days) was also evaluated in another phase II study on 71 cases of locally advanced NSCLC after induction with 2 cycles of cisplatin/docetaxel (Hallqvist et al., 2011). Toxicity was lower tha for most schedules with concurrent chemoradiotherapy. Esophagitis grade 1–2 occurred in 72% of patients, grade 3 in 1.4%. Skin reactions grade 1–2 occurred in 74% of patients and grade 3 in 4.2%. The median overall survival time was 17 months. The NEAR monocentric phase II trial enrolled 30 patients with locally advanced NSCLC who were treated with concomitant cetuximab and radiotherapy (Jensen et al., 2011). The overall response rate was 63%, partial remission occurred in 19/30 patients. The median progression-free survival time was 8.5 months and the median overall survival time was 19.5 months. The treatment was well tolerated with only mild toxicity (4 grade ≥ 3 pneumonitis). A phase II trial conducted by the Radiation Therapy Oncologic Group assessed a combination of cetuximab, chemotherapy and radiation (Blumenschein et al., 2008). Patients were given cetuximab every week and chemoradiotherapy (63 Gy in 35 fractions) was started during the second week, with weekly carboplatin/paclitaxel. The median survival time for the 87 evaluable patients was 22.7 months and the response rate was 62%. Adverse events related to treatment included 20% grade 4 hematological toxicities, 8% grade 3 cases of esophagitis, and 7% grade 3 to 4 cases of pneumonitis. There were five grade 5 events. The combination of cetuximab with chemoradiotherapy gave promising results, better than any previously reported by the Radiation Therapy Oncology Group.

Another schedule with carboplatin and pemetrexed was evaluated by Govindan et al. (Govindan et al. 2011). Patients with locally advanced NSCLC, including squamous carcinoma, were given carboplatin/pemetrexed every 21 days for four cycles and radiation therapy (70 Gy in 35 fractions) (arm A) or the same treatment plus cetuximab administered concurrent only with radiation therapy (arm B). The patients in both arms were given up to four cycles of pemetrexed as consolidation therapy. The the median failure-free survival times for the 101 eligible patients were 12.6 months in arm A and 12.3 months for those in arm B. The 18-month overall survival rates were 58% in arms A and 54% in arm B. The median overall survival times were 21.2 in arm A and 25.2 in arm B. The toxicities observed were consistent with the toxicities associated with concurrent chemoradiotherapy. These promising results need to be confirmed in further studies. No statistical difference was observed, probably due to the lack of power, and small number of patients.

Future directions: A phase III trial that is in progress will compare carpolatin/paclitaxel followed by radiotherapy to cetuximab and concurrent chemotherapy followed by radiotherapy in locally advanced NSCLC. Results are not expected before 2014 (National Cancer Institute, NCT00533949).

Table 10. Main NSCLC clinical trials of cetuximab combined with radiation. Gy: Gray; PC: carboplatin/paclitaxel

Authors	Drugs	Patients	Response rate	Toxicity
Phase I Hughes et al., 2008	platinum-based chemotherapy followed by cetuximab/radiation (64 Gy/32 fractions/45 days)	n=12		1 grade 2 skin reaction 1 grade 3 pneumonitis
Phase II Jatoi et al., 2010	Cetuximab + radiation (60 Gy/30 fractions/45 days)	n=57 elderly patients	PFS: 7.2 months OS: 15.1 months	Any Grade ≥3 adverse events in 31 patients
Phase II Hallqvist et al., 2011	Cetuximab + radiation (68 Gy/35 fractions/49 days)	n=71	OS: 17 months	Grade ≥3 oesophagite (1.4%)
Phase II Jensen et al., 2011	Cetuximab + radiation	n=30	Response rate 63% PFS: 8.5 months OS: 19.5 months	4 grade ≥ 3 pneumonitis
Phase II Blumenschein et al., 2008	Cetuximab + PC+ radiation (63 Gy in 35 fractions)	n=87	Response rate 62% OS: 22.7 months	8% grade ≥ 3 esophagitis, and 7% grade ≥ 3 pneumonitis
Phase II Govindan et al. 2011	Arm A: PC + radiation (70 Gy in 35 fractions) Arm B: Arm A + cetuximab	n=101	PFS: Arm A= 12.6 months Arm B= 12.3 months OS: Arm A= 21.2 months Arm B= 25.2 months	

2.2.2.4.5. Cetuximab and Predictive Markers

The clinical trials indicate that NSCLC patients respond well to cetuximab while others will not. The principal challenge is to discover predictive markers of the response of NSCLC to cetuximab. Cetuximab is only active on those patients with colorectal cancer with wild type *KRAS* (Allegra et al., 2009). The EGFR mutation is associated with a better response in lung adenocarcinoma patients treated with gefitinib than those treated with standard chemotherapy, and assays of EGFR mutations are now required before gefitinib is prescribed for lung adenocarcinomas (Maemondo et al., 2010).

BMS099, a large phase III clinical trial was carried out on 676 chemotherapy-naïve patients with advanced NSCLC of any histology or EGFR status. Their EGFR and KRas profiles were evaluated before they were assigned to treatment with paclitaxel/carboplatin with or without cetuximab (Khambata-Ford et al., 2010; Lynch et al., 2005). Tumor samples were available from 225 randomly assigned patients and biomarkers included K-Ras and EGFR mutations were analysed by direct sequencing, EGFR protein by immunohistochemistry (IHC), and EGFR gene copy number by fluorescent in situ hybridization (FISH). The progression free survival times of patients with KRas wild type treated with cetuximab (5.1 months) or without (5.3 months) were similar. The progression free survival time of patients with KRas mutations who were given cetuximab plus paclitaxel/carboplatin was twice as long (5.6 months) as that of patients given chemotherapy alone (2.8 months), but the difference was not statistically different. The overall survival times of wild type KRas patients treated with cetuximab (9.7 months) or without (9.9 months) were also similar. The overall survival times of patients with KRas mutations given cetuximab were longer (16.8 months) than those of patients not given cetuximab (10.8 months), but the difference was not statistically significant. KRas mutations were found in only 17% of the evaluable patients, which may explain why the difference was not statistically significant. EGFR mutations were found in 10% (17/166) of patients, while 89% (131/148) of patients were EGFR positive by IHC, and 52% (54/104) of patients were FISH positive. The progression-free survival and overall survival times of these sub-groups, excluding those who were FISH positive, were similar. The overall survival times of the FISH-positive patients treated with chemotherapy alone was statistically longer (12.5 months) than that of patients treated with cetuximab (8.6 months), but the progression-free survival times were similar (5.4 months). This overall survival times is probably influenced by the second line therapy and we think that patients given chemotherapy alone in first line were probably given EGFR TKI as the second line, which could explain this difference. Another clinical trial assessed EGFR FISH in 76 patients treated with paclitaxel/carboplatin with or without cetuximab for up to 4 cycles, followed by cetuximab for up to 1 year for overall patients (Hirsch et al., 2008). The median progression-free survival time of the patients with FISH-positive tumors was statistically longer (6 months) than that of FISH-negative patients (3 months). The median overall survival time was also longer (15 months) than that of the FISH-negative patients (7 months). Further studies are needed to clarify the relationship between EGFR status and the response to cetuximab.

A post-hoc analysis of the FLEX study collected and quantified the immunohistochemical EGFR activity in tumors (Pirker et al., 2012). Tumour EGFR immunohistochemistry data were available for 1121/1125 patients (99·6%). Of these, 345 (31%) patients had high EGFR activity and 776 (69%) had low EGFR activity. The overall survival time of the high EGFR patients treated with chemotherapy plus cetuximab was statistically significantly longer (12·0 months) than that of the high EGFR patients given chemotherapy alone (9.6 months). However the progression-free survival times of the two groups were similar (5 months for chemotherapy plus cetuximab and 4.6 months in chemotherapy alone). Toxicity was not increased in the high EGFR patients. Prospective studies are needed to confirm these results.

Skin rash is the most adverse events observed with cetuximab treatment. Another post-hoc analysis of the FLEX study compared skin rash at first cycle was to survival time (Gatzemeier et al., 2011). The overall survival time of patients in the chemotherapy plus cetuximab group with a first cycle rash was significantly longer (15.0 months) than that of patients in the same treatment group with no first-cycle rash (8.8 months). There were also significant associations between progression-free survival times and first cycle rash: 5.4 months for patients treated with chemotherapy plus cetuximab and 4·3 months those given chemotherapy alone. The overall survival for patients without first-cycle rash (8.8 months) was similar to that of patients given chemotherapy alone (10.3 months). These results should be confirmed in a prospective study.

2.2.3. Anti-EGFR: Matuzumab

Matuzumab is a humanized IgG1 monoclonal antibody targeting EGFR with high affinity, competitively blocking natural ligands and thus inhibiting downstream EGFR-mediated signaling (Kim et al., 2004;. Its affinity for EGFR is a little lower than that of cetuximab but, matuzumab has a longer half-life (6–8 days) than cetuximab and does not induce autoantibodies, a known problem with chimeric and murine antibodies (Vanhoefer et al., 2004; Socinski et al., 2007). Matuzumab has antitumor activity on preclinical xenografts and cell line models (Burger A, et al., 2003). A phase I escalating dose study on 18 NSCLC patients given weekly increasing doses of matuzumab (100, 200, 400 or 800 mg) followed by 175 mg/m2 paclitaxel every 3 weeks found that the maximum planned matuzumab dose of 800 mg was below the maximum tolerate dose (Table 11) (Kollmannsberger et al., 2006).

The most frequent matuzumab-related side-effect was a grade 1/2 acneiform skin rash in 14 patients. Pharmacokinetics parameters were estimated. Peak serum concentrations were generally achieved within 1–4 h after starting infusion. The mean Cmax values for weekly doses of 100 - 800 mg were 33.5 - 248.6 μg/ml. The terminal elimination t1/2 was not constant and increased from 38.7 h at 100 mg to 137.6 h at 800 mg. Of 18 patients, three achieved a partial response and one a complete response (overall response rate 22%).

An additional 8 patients were added to this clinical trial to determine molecular predictive factors for response to mastuzumab (Schittenhelm et al., 2009). EGFR expression and the KRAS mutation status seemed to predict a clinical response to matuzumab. A group of 148 NSCLC patients were recently given 500 mg/m^2 pemetrexed every 3 weeks alone (n = 50), or combined with matuzumab (either 800 mg/week; n = 51, or 1600 mg every 3 weeks; n = 47) (Schiller et al., 2010).

The objective response rate for the pooled matuzumab groups was 11%, while that of the pemetrexed alone was 5%, but the difference was not statistically significant. All the patients who responded had tumors containing EGFR, except for one patient in the pemetrexed alone group. The objective response rate for patients given weekly matuzumab was 16%; it was 2% for those given matuzumab every 3 weeks. The overall survival of patients given matuzumab weekly (12.4 months) tended to be better than that of patients given matuzumab every 3 weeks (5.9 months); it was 7.9 months for patients on pemetrexed alone. The safety profile was acceptable. The most common grade 3/4 adverse event was neutropenia. We have been unable to find any phase III trial published or registered on the internet (http://clinicaltrials.gov).

2.2.4. Anti-EGFR: Nimotuzumab

Nimotuzumab, a monoclonal antibody targeting anti-EGFR, was originally isolated as a mouse IgG2a antibody (R3) and humanized by grafting its complementarity-determining regions (CDRs) onto a human IgG1 gene (Mateo et al., 1997). The R3 mAb was humanized to reduce its human immunogenicity and slow clearance from the body. The binding affinity of nimotuzumab to EGFR is similar to that of EGF, but it is 10-fold less than competing mAbs, cetuximab, and panitumumab (Boland et al., 2010).

In vitro, nimotuzumab inhibited the EGF-induced EGFR phosphorylation in a concentration-dependent manner in H292 cells (which have a high concentration of surface EGFR), whereas it did not substantially affect this phosphorylation in H460 or H1299 cells (both of which have a low surface concentrations of EGFR) (Akashi et al., 2008).

It enhanced the cytotoxic effect of radiation in H292 cells but not in H460 or H1299 cells. In the H460 xenograft model, tumour growth was inhibited by radiation alone but not by nimotuzumab alone, and nimotuzumab did not enhance the effect of radiation. In contrast, both radiation and nimotuzumab inhibited the growth of tumours formed by H292 cells and their combined treatment substantially delayed tumour growth; the combination also inhibited the growth of H292 xenografts.

Table 11. Main NSCLC clinical trials of anti-HER antibodies excluding cetuximab. PC: carboplatin/paclitaxel; Cis/Gem: Cipslatin/Gemcitabine; PFS: progression free survival; OS: Overall survival

Authors	Drugs	Patients	Response rate	Toxicity
Phase II Schiller et al., 2010	Arm A: Pemetrexed alone Arm B: Pemetrexed + Matuzumab weekly Arm C: Pemetrexed + Matuzumab every 3 weeks	n=148	Objective response rate Arm A = 5% Arm B + C = 11% OS: Arm A= 7.9 months Arm B= 12.4 months Arm C= 5.9	Most grade 3 adverse event was neutropenia
Phase II Bebb et al., 2011	Nimotuzumab + radiation (30 or 36 Gy in 3 Gy fractions)	n=18	Objective response rate 66% PFS: 4.2 months OS: 14.3 months	Any Grade ≥3 adverse events in 31 patients
Phase II Blumenschein et al., 2010	Arm A: PC + motesanib Arm B: Panitumumab + motesanib Arm C: Arm B + PC	n=45	objective response rate: Arm A=17% Arm B=0% Arm C=17%	
Phase I Kuenen et al., 2010	Necitumumab alone	n=60 including 4 NSCLC patients	Response rate = 0% in NSCLC	
Phase II Lara et al., 2003	Trastuzumab or docetaxel followed by trastuzumab+docetaxel	n=13	PFS: 4.3 months OS: 5.7 months	
Phase II Clamon et al., 2004	Trastuzumab alone	n=209	Response rate 5% PFS: 2.6 months OS: 5.3 months	One treatment-related death due to pulmonary toxicity
Phase II Langer et al., 2005	Trastuzumab + PC	n=139	Response rate 25% PFS= 3.3 months OS= 10.1 months	grade ≥ 3 neutropenia 57%.
Phase II Zinner et al., 2004	Trastuzumab + Cis/Gem	n=21	PFS= 8.5 months OS= 16.7 months	
Phase II Gatzemeier et al., 2004	Arm A: Trastuzumab + Cis/Gem Arm B: Cis/Gem	n=103	Response rate Arm A=36% Arm B=41% PFS Arm A=6.1 months Arm B= 7 months	
Phase II Herbst et al., 2007	Pertuzumab + Erlotinib	n=43	PFS=1.5 months	4 Grade 3/4 adverse events

A phase I clinical trial included 18 advanced NSCLC patients who were given nimotuzumab weekly (100, 200 or 400 mg) with radiation (30 or 36 Gy in 3 Gy fractions) for

8 weeks (Bebb et al., 2011). Nimotuzumab was continued for patients who responded or whose disease stabilized; it was given every other week starting from week 10 until progression or toxicity became unmanageable. The most commonly reported adverse events were fatigue, anorexia, chills, pain and hypophosphatemia (grades 1 to 2 in most patients). There were no reports of severe skin or allergic toxicity. The maximum tolerated dose was not reached. The objective response rate was 66 % and the disease control rate was 94.0%. The median progression-free survival time was 4.2 months and the median overall survival time was 14.3 months. A similar clinical trial was conducted on 15 Korean patients who were given a combination of nimotuzumab and radiation. One patient given 200 mg nimotuzumab developed grade 4 pneumonia with neutropenia. No other patients reached dose limiting toxicity.

Other clinical trials are in progress. The safety of chemotherapy (cisplatin/docetaxel) combined with nimotuzumab is currently being assessed in a phase I trial (Biotech Pharmaceutical Co., Ltd, NCT00985998). The progression-free survival of NSCLC patients treated with a combination of nimotuzumab and docetaxel was also evaluated (Biotech Pharmaceutical Co., Ltd, NCT00983047). The results of both of these studies were expected in 2010, but we are not aware of any published data. The combination of gefitinib/nimotuzumab has been compared to gefitinib alone in NSCLC patients and results are due to be published in June 2012 (Byoung Chul Cho, NCT01498562). Finally, another study has compared the combination of nimotuzumab/liposomal paclitaxel/carboplatin to chemotherapy alone in NSCLC patients (Biotech Pharmaceutical Co., Ltd, NCT01393080). The results of this trial are expected in 2014.

2.2.5. Anti-EGFR: Panitumumab

Panitumumab is a fully humanized IgG2 anti-EGFR monoclonal antibody that binds with a high affinity (Heymach et al., 2006). Panitumumab inhibited the ligand-dependent autophosphorylation of EGFR in mutant EGFR-bearing CHO and NSCLC cells *in vitro* (A549) (Freeman et al., 2009). And panitumumab alone or combined with cisplatin inhibited the growth of tumors in NCI-H1975 and NCIH1650 xenograft models significantly more than the control treatment (human IgG2). Panitumumab plus docetaxel had greater antitumor activity in xenograft models than did panitumumab alone. Panitumumab does not induce an ADCC because it is an IgG2 antibody. The safety, pharmacokinetics and anti-tumor activity of panitumumab was evaluated in a phase I trial on 96 patients with various solid malignancies, including 14 with NSCLC (Weiner et al., 2008). The serum panitumumab concentrations of patients given 2.5 mg/kg weekly, 6.0 mg/kg every 2 weeks, and 9.0 mg/kg every 3 weeks were similar. The maximum tolerated dose was not reached. None of the NSCLC patients had a partial response and only 5 had a stable disease. Panitumumab in association with motesanib, a small-molecule antagonist of vascular endothelial growth factor receptors 1, 2, and 3, platelet-derived growth factor receptor, and Kit was assessed recently in a clinical trial (Blumenschein et al., 2010). The 45 patients with unresectable NSCLC were given sequentially escalating oral doses of motesanib plus carboplatin/paclitaxel (arm A), or motesanib plus panitumumab (arm B), or motesanib plus panitumumab plus carboplatin/paclitaxel (arm C). The maximum tolerated dose of motesanib was 125 mg once daily. The objective response rates were 17% in arm A, 0% in arm B, and 17% in arm C.

Various clinical trials testing panitumumab in NSCLC are currently in progress. A trial to test pre-operative chemoradiotherapy with or without panitumumab in advanced NSCLC patients is currently recruiting participants (National Cancer Institute, NCT00979212). The safety of the pemetrexed/carboplatin/panitumumab combination is also being evaluated in another phase II trial (Amgen, NCT01042288). Finally, two clinical trials designed to evaluate the response rate to carboplatin/vinorelbin/panitumumab as first line therapy and the progression-free survival time for cisplatin/pemetrexed with or without panitumumab are in progress (Vejle Hospital, NCT01038037; Gesellschaft fur Medizinische Innovation – Hamatologie und Onkologie mbH, NCT01088620).

2.2.6. Anti-EGFR: Necitumumab

Necitumumab is a fully human IgG1 monoclonal antibody that targets the EGFR extracellular domain III (Dienstmann et al., 2011). Its affinity for EGFR is similar to that of cetuximab (Li et al., 2005). Necitumumab combined with cisplatin and gemcitabine was tested in two mouse xenograft models of NSCLC (A549 and NCI-H1650) (Prewett et al., 2009).

Necitumumab plus chemotherapy inhibited the growth of xenografted tumors significantly better than either therapy alone. Necitumumab plus cisplatin plus gemcitabine caused the partial regression of A549 tumors in 33% of treated mice, but no regression was seen in mice given any one of the treatments. A group of 60 patients with advanced solid malignancies were treated with 100 to 1,000 mg of necitumumab in a phase I trial (Kuenen et al., 2010). Treatment was given every week (n=29 including 1 patient with NSCLC) or every 2 weeks (n=31 including 3 patients with NSCLC). Two patients given 1,000 mg every 2 weeks experienced dose-limiting toxicities (DLT; grade 3 headache), one patient also had grade 3 nausea and vomiting. The maximum tolerated dose was 800 mg. Toxicity was similar on both schedules.

Necitumumab had saturable elimination and nonlinear pharmacokinetics. Its half-life was approximately 7 days when given at 800 mg (both arms). Two patients had a partial response, one with melanoma and the other with colorectal cancer. The recommended dose of necitumumab for further clinical development is 800 mg weekly or every 2 weeks. Necitumumab is being evaluated combined with cisplatin and gemcitabine in a phase III trial of advanced NSCLC (NCT00981058). In this randomized, multicenter, open-label trial, NSCLC patients will be treated with either necitumumab and gemcitabine-cisplatin or chemotherapy alone as first-line therapy. Chemotherapy is continued for a maximum of six cycles and necitumumab until the disease progresses or toxicity becomes intolerable. The primary endpoint will be the overall survival time. Preliminary results will be presented in September 2013. Another phase III study comparing pemetrexed/cisplatin/necitumumab to chemotherapy alone in chemo-naive NSCLC was stopped prematurely (Parexe, NCT00982111) According to the press release from the company, the independent Data Monitoring Committee (DMC) decided that new or recently enrolled patients should stop treatment because of safety concerns about thromboembolisms (blood clots) in the experimental arm of the study (Press Release: Lilly. Bristol-Myers Squibb, 2011)

2.2.7. Anti-HER2: Trastuzumab

Trastuzumab is a humanized monoclonal antibody IgG1 directed against the Her2 receptor. It is widely used in breast cancer but clinical results in NSCLC are less encouraging.

2.2.7.1. Preclinical Studies

The effects of trastuzumab alone, and trastuzumab/gemcitabine in combination were evaluated *in vitro* on 4 NSCLC cell lines (H322, A549, H460 and Calu-3) and 2 breast cancer cell lines (Hirsh et al., 2002). Trastuzumab alone inhibited the growth of all the cell lines expressing HER2 and the inhibitory effect was correlated with the concentration of HER2 protein at the cell surface. Trastuzumab and gemcitabine acted in and the degree of synergy was not directly correlated with the concencentration of HER2 protein at the cell surface. Trastuzumab seemed to have greater antitumor activity against NSCLC xenografts than against breast cancer xenografts.

2.2.7.2. Clinical Studies

Giving trastuzumab after adjuvant chemotherapy increased the disease-free survival time of patients with HER2-positive breast cancers (Piccart-Gebhart et al., 2005). But the results are less encouraging in lung cancer, probably due to the heterogeneity of HER2 overproduction.

A phase II trial on 69 patients with NSCLC (33 men, 36 women) who were screened immunohistochemically for HER2 overproduction found that only 13 (19%) had a HER2-positive disease (Lara et al., 2003). Patients with HER2-positive tumors were initially given single-agent trastuzumab or docetaxel for 2 treatment cycles. All the patients were then given trastuzumab plus docetaxel regardless of their response to the single agents. There was 1 partial response among the 9 patients given docetaxel alone. The overall outcomes to the sequence of a single agent followed by combination therapy were a partial response in 8% of cases, a stable disease in 23%, a progressive disease in 46%, and an unassessable disease in 23%. The event-free survival time was 4.3 months and the overall survival time was 5.7 months. The treatment was well tolerated. In another phase II trial, trastuzumab alone had poor anti-NSCLC tumor activity (Clamon et al., 2004). The 209 patients screened included 24 (11%) with tumors with a moderate or high HER-2 concentration. Only one patient had a partial response, and one patient suffered treatment-related pulmonary toxicity and died.

The combination of carboplatin/paclitaxel/trastuzumab was also assessed in a phase II trial on 139 advanced and metastatic NSCLC patients (Langer et al., 2005). Of these, 50 (36%) were HER-2/neu negative, 38 (27%) had low concentrations of HER-2, 31 (22%) had moderate concentrations and 13 (9%) had high HER-2 concentrations. Only 13 of the 52 assessable patients had an objective response. The incidence of grade ≥ 3 neutropenia was 57%. The median progression-free survival time was 3.3 months; the median survival time was 10.1 months, and the 1-year survival rate was 42%. Finally, 2 studies evaluated the combination of cisplatin/gemzar/trastuzumab for treating NSCLC. The first enrolled only 21 NSCLC patients with HER2 and 8 (38%) of them had a partial response (Zinner et al., 2004). The 1-year survival rate was 62% (13/21) and the median time to progression was 8.5 months. The other enrolled 103 NSCLC patients with HER2 overproduction and 51 were treated with trastuzumab plus gemcitabine–cisplatin, while 50 were given gemcitabine–cisplatin alone (Gatzemeier et al., 2004). The efficacy of the trastuzumab and control arms were similar, with response rates of 36% and 41%; median times to progression of 6.3 months and 7.2 months; and median progression-free survival times of 6.1 months and 7 months.

To the best of our knowledge, no phase III trial has been published or registered (http://clinicaltrials.gov).

2.2.8. HER dimerization inhibitors: Pertuzumab

Pertuzumab is a humanized monoclonal antibody that binds to the dimerization domain of HER2, which is distinct from the domain recognized by trastuzumab (Franklin et al., 2004). It is therefore a dimerization inhibiting mAb (Sakai et al., 2007). The *in vitro* antitumor activity of pertuzumab was assessed in NSCLC 11_18 cells that bear large amounts of HER2 and HER3. Heregulin (HRG)-α is a ligand of the HER3 receptor and EGF is the ligand of EGFR (HER1). Pertuzumab inhibited the HRG-α-dependent growth of 11_18 lung cancer cells inhibiting HRG-α-stimulated HER2/HER3 signaling. Treatment of Calu-3 NSCLC xenografts with pertuzumab or trastuzumab significantly inhibited tumor growth (Scheuer et al., 2009). A combination of trastuzumab and pertuzumab had a much greater antitumor activity than each agent alone. Erlotinib/pertuzumab combination therapy inhibited mouse Calu-3 NSCLC xenografts much better than the sum of each individual agent (Friess et al., 2005). A phase I clinical trial in which 43 NSCLC chemonaïve patients were treated with pertuzumab i.v. every 3 weeks found no responses (Herbst et al., 2007). The median progression-free survival time was 1.5 months. Of 22 patients who underwent F-18-fluorodeoxyglucose positron emission tomography, six (27.3%) with a metabolic response to pertuzumab had a statistically significant longer progression-free survival time than the 16 patients who had no metabolic response. Only 4 patients (9.3%) experienced a grade 3/4 adverse event judged related to pertuzumab. Lastly, a phase II clinical trial will assess the combination of erlotinib and pertuzumab in an estimated 70 patients with relapsed non-small cell lung cancer. The primary outcome is the response to F-18-fluorodeoxyglucose positron emission tomography (Roche Pharma AG, NCT00855894).

2.3. Antibodies against the Insulin Growth Factor (IGF) Pathway

2.3.1. IGF Pathway

The IGF system comprises circulating ligands (IGF-1, IGF-2 and insulin), multiple receptors (Rs), and a family of IGF binding proteins (IGFBPs 1–6) (Furstenberger et al. 2002). IGF-1R signaling is transduced via two main pathways: the RAS–RAF–MAP kinase pathway that predominantly stimulates cell proliferation, and the phosphoinositide-3 kinase (PI3 K)–Akt–mammalian target of rapamycin (mTOR) pathway that mainly mediates cell survival (Samani et al., 2007; Kawauchi et al. 2009; Giorgio et al. in press). The presence of IGF1-R is associated with shorter disease-free survival times in NSCLC patients (Nakagawa et al., 2012) and is a target for NSCLC treatment.

2.3.2. Anti-IGF1R Antibody: Figitumumab

Figitumumab (CP-751,871) is a fully human IgG2 monoclonal antibody that is specific for IGF1-R (Gualberto et al., 2010). It significantly inhibited the growth of EBC-1 xenografts, a model of squamous NSCLC, but not that of the A549 or H460 cell models (Gualberto et al. 2009). Figitumumab also enhanced the antitumor activity of a variety of anticancer therapies, including erlotinib, cisplatin, and paclitaxel (Cohen et al., 2005; Gualberto et al., 2009). A phase I clinical trial on 35 patients with advanced NSCLC given paclitaxel/carboplatin /figitumumab (0.05–20 mg/kg) every 3 weeks for up to six cycles did nto reach the maximum tolerated dose and concentrations of bioactive IGF-1 seemed to influence the response to treatment, with objective responses in patients with a high baseline free IGF-1 (Karp et al., 2009b). A phase II study in which 151 NSCLC patients were randomly assigned to receive either paclitaxel/carboplatin/figitumumab (PCF) (10 to 20 mg/kg) or paclitaxel/carboplatin alone (PC) found that the combination treatment was well tolerated (Karp et al., 2009a). There was grade 3 to 4 hyperglycemia in 15% of patients treated with PCF and in 8% of those given PC. Over half (54%) of the patients treated with combination and 42% of those treated with chemotherapy alone had objective responses. Analysis of markers by objective response identified an association between the IGF1-R concentration and a partial response in squamous NSCLC patients treated with chemotherapy plus figitumumab (Gualberto et al., 2010). Baseline free IGF-1 concentration was correlated with the clinical benefit in NSCLC patients treated with figitumumab (Gualberto et al., 2011). Another phase I trial in which 46 patients, including 2 NSCLC patients, were treated with docetaxel and figitumumab did not reach the maximum tolerated dose (Molife et al., 2009). The pharmacokinetics of docetaxel/figitumumab were similar to those of docetaxel given alone. Four patients had a partial response but none of them had NSCLC. A phase III study in which NSCLC patients were given carboplatin/paclitaxel/figitumumab or chemotherapy alone was shut down early because of too many deaths linked to figitumumab therapy (Pfizer, NCT00596830). The results of the study indicated that the overall survival of patients given figitumumab plus chemotherapy (8.5 months) was worse than for those given chemotherapy alone (10.3 months) (http://www.ascopost.com/articles/november-2010/figitumumab-fails-to-improve-survival,-increases-toxicities,-in-first%E2%80%91line-treatment-of-patients-with-nsclc/). However, figitumumab/chemotherapy was associated with better overall survival than was chemotherapy alone in a subset of patients with high baseline circulating IGF1-R. A phase III trial that compared erlotinib/figitumumab and erlotinib alone as a second-line therapy for NSCLC patients was prematurely closed because there was no improvement in the progression-free survival time in intermediate analyses (Pfizer, NCT00673049).

2.3.3. Anti-IGF1-R: Dalotuzumab

Dalotuzumab (MK-0646 or h7C10) is a humanized IgG1 monoclonal antibody directed against IGF-1R that was selected on the basis of its specificity for IGF-1R rather than the insulin receptor. The average tumor volume in A549 xenograft mouse models at 6 weeks post-cell injection was reduced by 72% (Goetsch, et al., 2005). The capacities of vinorelbine alone and dalotuzumab alone to inhibit growth were similar. Dalotuzumab reduced the average tumor volume at 10 weeks post cell injection by 55% and vinorelbine reduced it by 51%. Combined therapy inhibited growth by 94% compared with control mice. Similar results were obtained with cetuximab plus dalotuzumab. A phase I trial was carried out on 80 patients with various cancers to assess the safety of dalotuzumab (Atzori et al., 2011). The number of patients with NSCLC was not given. Only 5 patients had grade ≥ 3 adverse events. Another phase I/IIa trial assessed the safety of erlotinib/dalotuzumab in previously treated NSCLC patients (Merck, NCT00654420). Results are expected soon. A phase II trial will compare pemetrexed/cisplatin/dalotuzumab with chemotherapy alone in chemoniave non-squamous NSCLC patients (Merck, NCT00799240). The primary endpoint will be the response rate. Finally, the progression-free survival of NSCLC patients treated with gemcitabine/carboplatin/dalotuzumab will be evaluated (National Cancer Institute, NCT00951444).

2.3.4. Cixitumumab

Cixitumumab (IMC-A12) is a fully human IgG1 monoclonal antibody which was engineered to selectively bind to the IGF-IR, thereby blocking ligand binding and signaling through downstream mitogen-activated protein kinase and phosphoinositide-3-kinase/AKT pathways (Burtrum et al., 2003). Cixitumumab had a good anti-tumor effect on H226 cells and moderate effect on A549 cells *in vitro* (Allen et al., 2005). A combination of anti-EGFR and anti-IGF1-R had a dramatically enhanced antitumor effect on H226 cells. A phase I/II trial on 18 patients with chemonaive advanced NSCLC who were treated with 150 mg/d erlotinib and 5 or 6 mg/kg cixutumumab every week or 15 mg/kg every 3 weeks found that 4 of the 6 patients given 6 mg/kg experienced dose-limiting toxicities (DLTs), while 1 of the 8 patients on 5 mg/kg experienced DLT and 3/8 patients still required a dose delay during cycle 1. 2/4 patients given 15 mg/kg every 21 days experienced DLTs (Weickhardt et al., 2012). The DLTs were a grade 3 rash or fatigue. The best response of 5 patients was a stable disease. A phase II trial that is still recruiting NSCLC participants will treat them with bevacizumab/carboplatin/paclitaxel with or without cixitumumab (National Cancer Institute, NCT00955305).

The primary endpoint will be the progression-free survival time. Another combination that is currently being tested is gemcitabine/cisplatin/cetuximab with or without cixitumumab (ImClone LLC, NCT00870870). Finally, erlotinib/cixitumumab was compared with erlotinib alone in a phase II trial (National Cancer Institute, NCT00778167).

2.3.5. Other Anti-IGF1-R Antibodies

2.3.5.1.BIIB022

BIIB022 is a fully human monoclonal IgG4 unglycosylated antibody that binds specifically to IGF-1R (Giorgio et al., in press). It is currently being assessed for treating lung cancer in a phase I trial combined with carboplatin/paclitaxel (Biogen Idec, NCT00970580).

2.3.5.2. RG1507

RG1507 is a fully human IgG1 monoclonal antibody directed against IGF-1R (Bagatel et al., 2010). The 172 NSCLC patients in a phase II clinical trial were given erlotinib plus placebo, or R1507 9 mg/kg weekly, or R1507 16 mg/kg intravenously once every 3 weeks as second-line therapy (Ramalingam et al., 2011). Grades 3 to 4 adverse events occurred in 37% of the patients on placebo, in, 44% of those on R1507 weekly, and in 48% of those on R1507 every 3 weeks.

The progression-free survival rates were 39%, 37%, and 44%, and the median overall survival times were 8.1, 8.1, and 12.1 months for the three groups, with statistically unsignificant hazard ratios. The 12-week progression-free survival rate in patients with the KRAS mutation was 36% given R1507 and only 0% for those on placebo. No clinical phase III trial has yet been registered.

2.3.5.3. Robatumumab

Robatumumab is a fully human IgG1 antibody directed against IGF1-R. We know of no clinical trial on NSCLC.

2.3.5.4. Ganitumab

Ganitumab is a fully human IgG1 monoclonal antibody directed against the human IGF1R (Beltran et al., 2011). It is currently being assessed in phase II clinical trials for use on NSCLC combined with carboplatin/paclitaxel or conatumumab (Amgen, NCT00807612; Amgen, NCT00819169).

2.4. Anti-CTLA-4 Antibodies

2.4.1. CTLA-4 in Lung Cancer

CTLA-4 is an immunoglobulin which is present on the surface of T cells. It binds to CD80 and CD86 on antigen-presenting cells. The CTLA4 on the surface of activated T-cells binds to B7, a costimulatory protein found on the surface of activated antigen-presenting cell, to send an inhibitory signal that stops T-cell activation, and this natural brake alters both downstream cytokine production and the cell-cycle machinery required for proliferation (Camacho et al., 2008). Failure of the immune system to recognize and eradicate tumor cells is believed to be a key mechanism in tumor development and recurrence (Holtan et al., 2011). Thus, blocking the CTLA-4-mediated termination signal with antibodies should prolong anti-tumor immune responses, resulting in enhanced tumor suppression. Two CTLA-4 blocking mAbs were tested on xenografts of RPCI-2E9 (human squamous cell carcinoma cells) and RPCI-9530 (human lung adenocarcinoma cells). They significantly enhanced the human lymphocyte-mediated tumor suppression in mice co-engrafted with autologous peripheral blood cells and tumor cells (Sabel et al., 2005).

2.4.2. Ipilumumab

Ipilimumab is a fully human IgG1 monoclonal antibody targeting CTLA-4 derived from transgenic mice. It is already approved by the FDA for treating metastatic melanomas. Iit is being evaluated in several clinical trials for use in NSCLC. One phase II trial will test ipilimumab plus paclitaxel as a maintenance treatment for NSCLC patients who did not progress after treatment with platinum-based chemotherapy (Bristol-Myers Squibb, NCT01471197). The primary end point is the overall survival rate. Another phase II study is treating NSCLC patients with alone or with carboplatin/paclitaxel plus concurrent or sequential ipilimumab (Bristol-Myers Squibb, NCT00527735). The preliminary results of this study are encouraging. Finally, a phase III trial has just started that compares carboplatin/paclitaxel/ ipilimumab to carboplatin/paclitaxel alone (Bristol-Myers Squibb, NCT01285609). The primary end point is overall survival.

2.4.3. Tremelimumab

Tremelimumab (CP-675,206) is a fully human IgG2 antibody specifically directed against CTLA-4 (Camacho et al., 2008). One phase II clinical trial was recently completed but results have not yet been published (Pfizer, NCT00312975). Tremelimumab was given to NSCLC patients immediately after first-line therapy and the primary end point was tht time until evidence of disease progression.

2.5. Anti-IL-6 Antibody: ALD518

Inflammation is associated with 15-20% of all deaths from cancer worldwide and contributes to fragility of cancer patients (Bayliss et al., 2011). The molecules involved in cancer-related inflammation include transcription factors (like NF-κB, signal transducers and activator of transcription 3 (STAT3)) and major inflammatory cytokines like IL-1β, IL-6, IL-23 and TNF-α (Mantovani et al., 2008). Data from several studies indicate that IL-6 plays an important role in NSCLC. Elevated plasma IL-6 concentrations were associated with a poor prognosis in NSCLC (Songur et al., 2004). ALD518 is a humanized IgG1 monoclonal antibody that binds with high affinity to human IL-6. The 124 NSCLC patients in a phase II study were given increasing doses of ALD518 (80 mg, 160 mg, 320 mg) (Rigas et al., 2010; Schuster et al., 2010). A total of 29 patients completed the treatment and were evaluated. Of the remaining patients, 38 failed to complete all the study visits, 52 patients died of progressive NSCLC and 5 patients withdrew due to adverse events. The toxicity-limiting dose was not reached. The hemoglobin concentration was higher in the patients given ALD518 than in the placebo group. Moreover, the pooled subjects treated with ALD518 lost statistically less of lean body mass (LBM).

2.6. TRAIL agonist Antibodies

The tumour necrosis factor-related apoptosis-inducing ligand (TRAIL), also known as Apo2L, is a member of the TNF ligand superfamily (Wiley et al, 1995, Pukac et al., 2005). It induces apoptosis in many cancer cell lines, with little or no effect on most normal cells (Wiley et al, 1995). TRAIL mediates apoptosis through two death receptors, TRAIL-receptor 1 (TRAIL-R1) and TRAIL-receptor 2 (TRAIL-R2). NSCLC patients have high tumor concentrations of TRAIL-R1 (in 67% to 99% of tumor biopsies) (Spierings et al., 2003; Cooper et al., 2008). TRAIL-R2 was detected in 82 % of NSCLC tumor biopsies.

2.6.1. Mapatumumab

Mapatumumab is a fully human agonist IgG1 monoclonal antibody specific for human TRAIL-R1. In vitro studies showed that H2122 NSCLC cell lines were very sensitive to mapatumumab, whereas H460 cells were moderately sensitive (Pukac et al., 2005). A combination of mapatumumab and cisplatin resulted in enhanced H460 cell killing, which was greater than the effect of each agent alone. H2122 xenografts treated with three weekly doses of mapatumumab (2.5 or 10 mg kg^{-1}) showed significant tumour regression even after a single injection. Tumour volume was reduced by approximately 50% on day 10 (4 days after the first injection) and by 97 % on day 25 with the 10 mg kg^{-1} dose. Treatment with mapatumumab or lexatumumab (TRAIL-R2 agonist described below) alone decreased the viability of H460 and H2122 cell in a dose-dependent manner, whereas A549, H441, H596, and H2347 cells were refractory to treatment with these antibodies (Luster et al., 2009). Bortezomib (100 nmol/L) significantly induced or enhanced the sensitivity of all NSCLC cell lines to mapatumumab and lexatumumab. The combination of mapatumumab or lexatumumab plus bortezomib rapidly generated an additive (H460 and H2122) or synergistic (A549, H596, H441, H2347) increase in cytotoxicity that killed around 100% of NSCLC cells treated with the highest concentration of antibody. The 32 patients with relapsed or refractory

Stage IIIB, or IV, or recurrent NSCLC were given 10 mg/kg mapatumumab IV every 21 days in a phase II trial (Greco et al., 2008). The mapatumumab was well tolerated, with no discontinuations due to adverse events. The most common adverse events reported, regardless of relationship, were fatigue, cough, nausea, dyspnea, constipation, and vomiting. None of the 32 patients treated showed a response according to the RECIST criteria. Nine patients (29%) had stable disease. In another phase II trial, 111 patients were randomly assigned to paclitaxel/carboplatin (Arm A), paclitaxel + carboplatin + 10 mg/kg mapatumumab (Arm B), or paclitaxel + carboplatin + 30 mg/kg mapatumumab (Arm C) (Von Pawel et al., 2010). The patients in Arms B and C could receive additional cycles of mapatumumab if ther was no disease progression.

Adding mapatumumab to chemotherapy did not improve the response rate (30.6% in A, 10.3% in B, and 36.1% in C) or the progression-free survival time (4.6 months in Arm A, 4.6 months in Arm B and 4.9 months in arm C). There was no evidence that mapatumumab exacerbated the toxicity associated with chemotherapy. No phase III trial has yet been organized.

2.6.2. Lexatumumab

Lexatumumab (HGS-ETR2) is an agonistic high-affinity IgG1 monoclonal antibody that binds to and activates TRAIL-R2 (Marini et al., 2006). Preclinical *in vitro* studies and studies on xenograft models showed that lexatumumab was active against various cancer cell lines, including NSCLC (Shimada et al., 2007; Zhang et al., 2007; Luster et al., 2009). Lexatumumab was clinically assessed in two phase I clinical trials that included various cancer patients. The first gave doses of lexatumumab from 0.1 to 20 mg/kg to 37 cancer patients (no NSCLC patients).

The 20 mg/kg dose was identified as the dose limting toxicity due to changes in serum amylase, transaminases, and bilirubin. The maximum tolerated dose was 10 mg/kg. To the best of our knowledge, no phase II trial has been registered. The 31 cancer patients, including 8 NSCLC, in the second trial were given one of 5 doses (0.1 to 10 mg/kg) of lexatumumab (Wakelee et al., 2007). One patient given 10 mg/kg experienced a possibly dose-related toxicity of grade 3 hyperamylasemia. Nine of the 31 patients achieved stable disease. The outcome of the NSCLC patients was not given.

2.6.3. Conatumumab

Conatumumab (AMG 655) is an agonistic high-affinity IgG1 monoclonal antibody that binds to and activates TRAIL-R2 (or death receptor 5) (Kaplan-Lefko et al., 2010). It inhibited the growth of NSCLC cell lines. The 37 cancer patients, including 7 with NSCLC, in a phase I clinical trial were given escalating doses of conatumumab (0.3, 1, 3, 10, or 20 mg/kg) intravenously every 2 weeks (Herbst et al., 2010). The 7 NSCLC patients were given 20 mg/kg every 2 weeks.

There were no dose-limiting toxicities. Only 3 patients had a grade 3 adverse event (fatigue and/or elevated lipase). The maximum tolerated dose was not reached. One patient with NSCLC (0.3 mg/kg) had a confirmed partial response at week 32 (38% reduction in tumor size), with a further reduction (48%) by week 96. This patient remains on conatumumab after 4.2 years with a sustained partial response.

2.6.4. Tigatuzumab

Tigatuzumab (TRA-8) is a humanized IgG1 monoclonal antibody directed against TRAIL-R2 that was selected from a series of anti-TRAIL-R2 monoclonal antibodies because of its specificity, ability to trigger apoptosis *in vitro* without the use of crosslinking reagents, and lack of toxicity to human hepatocytes (Ichikawa et al., 2001; Forero-Torres et al., 2010). Up to 8 mg/kg tigatuzumab was well tolerated by 17 cancer patients, but no NSCLC, in a phase I clinical trial. The maximum tolerated dose was not reached. No clinical trial on lung cancer patients is planned.

2.7. Bavituximab

As previously discussed, blood vessels are an attractive target in NSCLC therapeutic. Bavituximab is a vascular targeting agent with a unique mechanism of action (Daleke et al., 2003; Gerber et al., 2011). It is an unconjugated, chimeric IgG1 monoclonal antibody directed against the anionic phospholipids on the tumor endothelium. The principal target of bavituximab in most tissues, phosphatidylserine, is restricted to the internal surface of the cell membrane. But phosphatidylserine is exposed on the tumor vascular endothelium within solid tumors and particularly in hypoxic and stress situations (Jennewein et al., 2008).

Focal irradiation was used to increase the percentage of tumor vessels with exposed phosphatidylserine from 4% to 26% (He et al., 2007). Treating mice bearing A549 tumors with murin anti-phosphatidylserine plus focal radiation therapy inhibited tumor growth by 80% and was superior to radiation therapy or monoclonal antibody alone. The 26 patients with advanced solid malignancies (13 breast cancers, 4 colon cancer, 3 pancreatic cancer and 6 with other malignancies) that were progressing despite treatment in a phase I trial were given increasing doses of bavituximab, from 0.1 or 0.3 mg/kg bavituximab on days 0, 28, 35, and 42, or 1 and 3 mg/kg on days 0, 7, 14, and 21 (Gerber et al., 2011). The safety, pharmacokinetics, and tumor response were assessed. The maximum tolerated dose was not reached. Five patients suffered 6 serious adverse events, including one pulmonary embolism at 3 mg/kg, which was the only dose-limiting toxicity in the study. The half-life of bavituximab was 37 to 47 hours, with no accumulation following administration of multiple doses. There is no objective response for the 18 evaluable patients. Preliminary analysis of another phase II trial in which 49 Asian patients with untreated locally advanced or metastatic non-small cell lung cancer were given weekly doses of 3 mg/kg bavituximab intravenously until disease progression and up to 6 cycles of carboplatin and paclitaxel showed an overall response rate in the initial group of subjects of 11/21 (52.4%), with a clinical complete response in 4.8% and a partial response in 47.6% (Digumarti et al., 2010). The median progression-free survival time for the initial 21 patients treated was 6.2 month. The median overall urvival time is pending, as follow-up is continuing. Two phase II trials have been set up, one to compare carboplatin/paclitaxel to carboplatin/paclitaxel/bavituximab in chemonaive NSCLC patients and the other to compare docetaxel with docetaxel/bavituximab in previously treated NSCLC patients (Peregrine Pharmaceuticals, NCT01160601; Peregrine Pharmaceuticals, NCT01138163). The primary endpoint for both studies is the objective response rate.

2.8. Anti-NeuGcGM3: Racotumomab

Neu-glycolyl-containing gangliosides (NeuGcGM3) are glycolipids that are not normally components of the cytoplasmic membranes of humans. But Neu-glycolyl-containing gangliosides are overproduced by several human tumors (Malykh et al., 2001). Racotumomab is an anti-idiotype murine monoclonal antibody which reacts with NeuGc-containing gangliosides. A group of 71 previously treated NSCLC patients were given racotumomab in a phase II trial (Alfonso et al., 2007). No evidence of unexpected or serious adverse effects was reported. The median survival time of the 56 patients who entered the study with a partial response or a stable disease and with a PS 1 after the first line of chemo/radiotherapy was 11.50 months from starting treatment. In contrast, the median survival time calculated for patients who started treatment with progressive disease and/or a PS2 was 6.50 months.

2.9. Perspectives

2.9.1. Radioimmunoconjugates

As discussed in the first part, conjugation of mAbs with radionuclides may enhance their anti-tumor efficacy. Several radiolabeled antibodies are being evaluated for treating NSCLC. Two clinical trials showed that the toxicity of radiolabeled monoclonal antibody mCC49 directed against tumor-associated glycoprotein-72 (TAG-72) was acceptable, but the conjugate compound was no better than the unconjugated mAb (Robert et al., 2003; Forero et al., 2005). NSCLC patients were safely given Iodine-131-labeled tumor necrosis therapy (TNT) chimeric antibody by iv infusion, intratumorally or both (Yu et al., 2006). There were 2 partial responses among 16 patients given the compound iv, and 1 complete response and 1 partial response in the five patients given the compound by both routes. In the next few years, the side effects and best dose of radiolabeled cT84.66 monoclonal antibody, an antibody directed against CEA (Carcinoembryonic antigen), given together with radiation therapy and combination chemotherapy, will be assessed in patients with stage IIB, stage IIIA, or stage IIIB non-small cell lung cancer (National Cancer Institute, NCT00738452).

2.9.2. Drug-Conjugated Antibody

Immunoconjugates were assessed in two clinical studies on NSCLC patients. The first obtained some good results by giving SGN-15 (cBR96-doxorubicin conjugate) consisting of a chimeric murine monoclonal antibody that recognizes the Lewis Y antigen, conjugated to doxorubicin, to NSCLC patients (Ross et al., 2006). The overall survival rate at 18 months with SGN-15 was 18% and 8% with docetaxel alone. In the second trial, ABR-217620 (naptumomab estafenatox), a recombinant fusion protein consisting of a mutated variant of the superantigen staphylococcal enterotoxin E (SEA/E-120) linked to a Fab fragment that recognizes the tumor-associated antigen 5T4, was given alone or in combination with docetaxel (Borghaei et al., 2009). The treatment was well tolerated with evidence of immunological and antitumor activity.

2.9.3. Antibodies and Imaging

Only selected patients may profit from treatment with antibodies. Some authors have used radiolabeled antibodies in single photon-emission computed tomography (SPECT) and positron-emission tomography (PET) to select patients by visualizing the presence and activity of a specific antigen. The presence of antigen may predict antibody efficiency in selected patients (Xu et al., 2009). This promising method is still under evaluation for NSCLC. Biodistribution and PET studies on xenograft mouse models revealed a significantly high accumulation of ^{64}Cu-DOTA-trastuzumab in the NCI-H2170 tumor that overproduces Her2/neu 24 and 48 h post-injection (Paudyal et al., 2010).

Table 12. Therapeutic antibodies in NSCLC

	Target	Type	Immunoglobulin sub-class	Status in NSCLC
Bevacizumab	VEGF	Humanized	IgG1	Approved
Ramucirumab	VEGFR-2	Fully human	IgG1	Phase III
Ranibizumab	VEGF	Humanized	Fab	No clinical trial
Cetuximab	EGFR	Chimeric	IgG1	Phase III (Refusal)
Matuzumab	EGFR	Humanized	IgG1	Phase II
Nimotuzumab	EGFR	Humanized	IgG1	Phase II
Panitumumab	EGFR	Fully Human	IgG2	Phase II
Necitumumab	EGFR	Fully Human	IgG1	Phase III
Trastuzumab	HER2	Humanized	IgG1	Phase II
Pertuzumab	HER dimerization	Humanized	IgG1	Phase II
Figitumumab	IGF1-R	Fully human	IgG2	Phase III
Dalotuzumab	IGF1-R	Humanized	IgG1	Phase II
Cixitumumab	IGF1-R	Fully human	IgG1	Phase II
BIIB022	IGF1-R	Fully human	IgG4P	Phase I
Robatumumab	IGF1-R	Fully human	IgG1	No clinical trial
RG1507	IGF1-R	Fully human	IgG1	Phase II
Ipilimumab	CTLA-4	Fully human	IgG1	Phase III
Tremelimumab	CTLA-4	Fully human	IgG2	Phase II
ALD518	IL-6	Humanized	IgG1	Phase II
Mapatumumab	TRAIL-R1 (agonist	Fully human	IgG1	Phase II
Lexatumumab	TRAIL-R2 (agonist	Fully human	IgG1	Phase I
Conatumumab	TRAIL-R2 (agonist	Fully human	IgG1	Phase I
Tigatuzumab	TRAIL-R2 (agonist	Humanized	IgG1	Phase I
Racotumomab	NeuGcGM3	Murin	Ab2	Phase II
Bavituximab	Phosphatidylserine	Chimeric	IgG1	Phase II

2.9.4. Engineered mAbs

The simultaneous blockade of several antigens may enhance the anti-tumor effects of mAbs. Bi-specific mAbs with two different antigen binding sites have been developed for that purpose. Catumaxomab is a trifunctional monoclonal antibody (anti-EpCAM x anti-CD3) that interacts with three different cells types, tumor cells through the epithelial cell adhesion molecule (EpCAM) antigen, T-cells through the CD3 antigen and immune cell effectors through their FcγRs (Linke et al., 2010). Catumaxomab exerts its anti-tumor effects via T-cell-mediated lysis, ADCC, and phagocytosis via recruitment of FcγR-positive immune effector cells. It was approved in 2009 in Europe for the i.p. treatment of malignant ascites in patients with EpCAM-positive carcinomas where standard therapy is not available or no longer feasible. The phase I study by Sebastian et al. showed that catumaxomab could be delivered as a single intravenous 5 g infusion to patients who had been premedicated with 40 mg dexamethasone. The survival results seemed encouraging, although survival analysis was not the primary endpoint (Sebastian et al., 2007).

Conclusion

NSCLC is a cancer with a particularly poor prognosis that is generally refractory to anti-cancer treatments. Monoclonal antibodies offer new promising ways of treating NSCLC. Only one antibody, bevacizumab, is presently approved for NSCLC, but the progression-free survival time is short. Another mAb, cetuximab, was evaluated in several clinical trials and showed a small increase of overall survival in combination with chemotherapy. However, the FDA and the EMEA considered the therapeutic benefit insufficient and refused to approve cetuximab for treating NSCLC. At first glance, the results for NSCLC are somewhat disappointing, in contrast to the benefits obtained with mAb treatments in other solid tumors, such as breast and colon cancers. However, we believe this is only the visible part of the iceberg. The first steps towards treating NSCLC with therapeutic mAbs have been taken. Research and development of mAbs and derived compounds are a great challenge for both industry and academic institutions and countless possibilities remain to be explored. As proof, many mAb that have been approved for other cancers and new mAbs are being clinically evaluated for use with NSCLC. Cetuximab and anti-EGFR mAbs have not yet been abandoned as NSCLC treatments. Indeed, cetuximab is currently being tested in combination with radiation in clinical trials. New anti-cancer targets are being discovered every year and mAb technology to engineer more efficient biologics continues to evolve. Thus, the development of monoclonal antibodies clearly marks the start of a new era in NSCLC treatment, although there is still a long way to go before those "magic bullets" find their optimal target in lung cancer.

Acknowledgment

This publication was funded by the French National Research Agency under the program "Investissements d'avenir" Grant Agreement LabEx MAbImprove: ANR-10-LABX-53. It was also supported by the "fond de dotation en santé respiratoire", "Cancéropôle Grand Ouest," "Région Centre" and "Association régionale d'aide aux insuffisants respiratoires."

The English text was edited by Dr Owen Parkes.

For more information regarding ongoing clinical trials in NSCLC and cited in the book chapter, you could refer to http//:clinicaltrials.gov.

References

Adjei AA, Mandrekar SJ, Dy GK, Molina JR, Adjei AA, Gandara DR, et al. Phase II trial of pemetrexed plus bevacizumab for second-line therapy of patients with advanced non-small-cell lung cancer: NCCTG and SWOG study N0426. *J. Clin. Oncol.* 2010 févr 1;28(4):614–9.

Akashi Y, Okamoto I, Iwasa T, Yoshida T, Suzuki M, Hatashita E, et al. Enhancement of the antitumor activity of ionising radiation by nimotuzumab, a humanised monoclonal antibody to the epidermal growth factor receptor, in non-small cell lung cancer cell lines of differing epidermal growth factor receptor status. *Br. J. Cancer.* 2008 févr 26;98(4):749–55.

Alberti et al. Chemotherapy in non-small cell lung cancer: a meta-analysis using updated data on individual patients from 52 randomised clinical trials. Non-small Cell Lung Cancer Collaborative Group. *BMJ.* 1995 oct 7;311(7010):899–909.

Alfonso S, Diaz RM, de la Torre A, Santiesteban E, Aguirre F, Pérez K, et al. 1E10 anti-idiotype vaccine in non-small cell lung cancer: experience in stage IIIb/IV patients. *Cancer Biol. Ther.* 2007 déc;6(12):1847–52.

Amgen. Sarah Cannon Research Institute. Carboplatin, pemetrexed, and panitumumab in patients with advanced non-squamous K-ras wild type NSCLC. In: ClinicalTrials.gov [Internet]. Bethesda (MD): National Library of Medicine (US). 2000- [cited 2012 Feb 28]. Available from: http://clinicaltrials.gov/show/NCT01042288 NLM Identifier NCT01042288

Amgen. Phase 1b/2 study of AMG 479 in combination with paclitaxel and carboplatin for 1st line treatment of advanced squamous non-small cell lung cancer. In: ClinicalTrials.gov [Internet]. Bethesda (MD): National Library of Medicine (US). 2000- [cited 2012 Feb 28]. Available from: http://clinicaltrials.gov/show/NCT00807612 NLM Identifier NCT00807612

Amgen. AMG 655 in combination with AMG 479 in advanced, refractory solid tumors. In: ClinicalTrials.gov [Internet]. Bethesda (MD): National Library of Medicine (US). 2000- [cited 2012 Feb 28]. Available from: http://clinicaltrials.gov/show/NCT00819169 NLM Identifier: NCT00819169

Atzori F, Tabernero J, Cervantes A, Prudkin L, Andreu J, Rodríguez-Braun E, et al. A phase I pharmacokinetic and pharmacodynamic study of dalotuzumab (MK-0646), an anti-insulin-like growth factor-1 receptor monoclonal antibody, in patients with advanced solid tumors. *Clin. Cancer Res.* 2011 oct 1;17(19):6304–12.

Azinovic I, DeNardo GL, Lamborn KR, Mirick G, Goldstein D, Bradt BM, et al. Survival benefit associated with human anti-mouse antibody (HAMA) in patients with B-cell malignancies. *Cancer Immunol. Immunother.* 2006 déc;55(12):1451–8.

Azzoli CG, Temin S, Aliff T, Baker S Jr, Brahmer J, Johnson DH, et al. 2011 Focused Update of 2009 American Society of Clinical Oncology Clinical Practice Guideline Update on Chemotherapy for Stage IV Non-Small-Cell Lung Cancer. *J. Clin. Oncol.* 2011 oct 1;29(28):3825–31.

Bagatell R, Herzog CE, Trippett TM, Grippo JF, Cirrincione-Dall G, Fox E, et al. Pharmacokinetically guided phase 1 trial of the IGF-1 receptor antagonist RG1507 in children with recurrent or refractory solid tumors. *Clin. Cancer Res.* 2011 févr 1;17(3):611–9.

Bankhead. Study Dissects GI Risk of Bevacizumab. Clinical Oncology 2011 june 2011;06. http://www.clinicaloncology.com/ViewArticle.aspx?d=Solid+Tumorsandd_id=148andi=December+2011andi_id=799anda_id=19795.

Baselga J, Pfister D, Cooper MR, Cohen R, Burtness B, Bos M, et al. Phase I studies of anti-epidermal growth factor receptor chimeric antibody C225 alone and in combination with cisplatin. *J. Clin. Oncol.* 2000 févr;18(4):904–14.

Bayliss TJ, Smith JT, Schuster M, Dragnev KH, Rigas JR. A humanized anti-IL-6 antibody (ALD518) in non-small cell lung cancer. *Expert Opin. Biol. Ther.* 2011 déc;11(12):1663–8.

Bebb G, Smith C, Rorke S, Boland W, Nicacio L, Sukhoo R, et al. Phase I clinical trial of the anti-EGFR monoclonal antibody nimotuzumab with concurrent external thoracic radiotherapy in Canadian patients diagnosed with stage IIb, III or IV non-small cell lung cancer unsuitable for radical therapy. *Cancer Chemother. Pharmacol.* 2011 avr;67(4):837–45.

Belani CP, Schreeder MT, Steis RG, Guidice RA, Marsland TA, Butler EH, et al. Cetuximab in combination with carboplatin and docetaxel for patients with metastatic or advanced-stage nonsmall cell lung cancer: a multicenter phase 2 study. *Cancer.* 2008 nov 1;113(9):2512–7.

Beltran PJ, Chung Y-A, Moody G, Mitchell P, Cajulis E, Vonderfecht S, et al. Efficacy of ganitumab (AMG 479), alone and in combination with rapamycin, in Ewing's and osteogenic sarcoma models. *J. Pharmacol. Exp. Ther.* 2011 juin;337(3):644–54.

Biogen Idec. A study of BIIB022 in combination with paclitaxel and carboplatin in subjects with non-small cell lung cancer. In: ClinicalTrials.gov [Internet]. Bethesda (MD): National Library of Medicine (US). 2000- [cited 2012 Feb 28]. Available from: http://clinicaltrials.gov/show/NCT00970580 NLM Identifier: NCT00970580

Biotech Pharmaceutical Co., Ltd. Nimotuzumab in combination with cisplatin and docetaxel for patients with advanced non-small cell lung cancer. In: ClinicalTrials.gov [Internet]. Bethesda (MD): National Library of Medicine (US). 2000- [cited 2012 Feb 28]. Available from: http://clinicaltrials.gov/show/NCT00985998 NLM Identifier: NCT00985998

Biotech Pharmaceutical Co., Ltd. Nimotuzumab plus docetaxel in chemotherapy-refractory/resistant patients with advanced non-small-cell lung cancer. In: ClinicalTrials.gov [Internet]. Bethesda (MD): National Library of Medicine (US). 2000- [cited 2012 Feb 28]. Available from: http://clinicaltrials.gov/show/NCT00983047 NLM Identifier: NCT00983047

Biotech Pharmaceutical Co., Ltd. Yanzhao, Tianjin Medical University Cancer Institute and Hospital. Nimotuzumab in combination with paclitaxel liposome and carboplatin (TP Regimen) for the advanced NSCLC patients. In: ClinicalTrials.gov [Internet]. Bethesda (MD): National Library of Medicine (US). 2000- [cited 2012 Feb 28]. Available from: http://clinicaltrials.gov/show/NCT01393080 NLM Identifier: NCT01393080

Blumenschein GR Jr, Paulus R, Curran WJ, Robert F, Fossella F, Werner-Wasik M, et al. Phase II study of cetuximab in combination with chemoradiation in patients with stage IIIA/B non-small-cell lung cancer: RTOG 0324. *J. Clin. Oncol.* 2011 juin 10;29(17):2312–8.

Blumenschein GR Jr, Reckamp K, Stephenson GJ, O'Rourke T, Gladish G, McGreivy J, et al. Phase 1b study of motesanib, an oral angiogenesis inhibitor, in combination with carboplatin/paclitaxel and/or panitumumab for the treatment of advanced non-small cell lung cancer. *Clin. Cancer Res.* 2010 janv 1;16(1):279–90.

Bogart JA, Govindan R. A randomized phase II study of radiation therapy, pemetrexed, and carboplatin with or without cetuximab in stage III non-small-cell lung cancer. *Clin Lung Cancer.* 2006 janv;7(4):285–7.

Boland W, Bebb G. The emerging role of nimotuzumab in the treatment of non-small cell lung cancer. *Biologics.* 2010;4:289–98.

Bonner JA, Harari PM, Giralt J, Azarnia N, Shin DM, Cohen RB, et al. Radiotherapy plus cetuximab for squamous-cell carcinoma of the head and neck. *N. Engl. J. Med.* 2006 févr 9;354(6):567–78.

Borghaei H, Alpaugh K, Hedlund G, Forsberg G, Langer C, Rogatko A, et al. Phase I dose escalation, pharmacokinetic and pharmacodynamic study of naptumomab estafenatox alone in patients with advanced cancer and with docetaxel in patients with advanced non-small-cell lung cancer. *J. Clin. Oncol.* 2009 sept 1;27(25):4116–23.

Borghaei H, Langer CJ, Millenson M, Ruth KJ, Litwin S, Tuttle H, et al. Phase II study of paclitaxel, carboplatin, and cetuximab as first line treatment, for patients with advanced non-small cell lung cancer (NSCLC): results of OPN-017. *J. Thorac. Oncol.* 2008 nov;3(11):1286–92.

Boulianne GL, Hozumi N, Shulman MJ. Production of functional chimaeric mouse/human antibody. *Nature.* 1984 déc 13;312(5995):643–6.

Bowman T, Garcia R, Turkson J, Jove R. STATs in oncogenesis. *Oncogene.* 2000 mai 15;19(21):2474–88.

Brennan FR, Morton LD, Spindeldreher S, Kiessling A, Allenspach R, Hey A, et al. Safety and immunotoxicity assessment of immunomodulatory monoclonal antibodies. *MAbs.* 2010 juin;2(3):233–55.

Bristol-Myers Squibb. Memorial Sloan-Kettering. Cancer Center Cetuximab in patients with lung adenocarcinoma receiving erlotinib that have developed "acquired resistance" to erlotinib. In: ClinicalTrials.gov [Internet]. Bethesda (MD): National Library of Medicine (US). 2000- [cited 2012 Feb 28]. Available from: http://clinicaltrials.gov/show/NCT 00716456 NLM Identifier: NCT00716456

Bristol-Myers Squibb. Safety and efficacy trial of ipilimumab versus pemetrexed in non-squamous non-small cell lung cancer. In: ClinicalTrials.gov [Internet]. Bethesda (MD): National Library of Medicine (US). 2000- [cited 2012 Feb 28]. Available from: http://clinicaltrials.gov/show/NCT01471197 NLM Identifier NCT01471197

Bristol-Myers Squibb. Phase II study for previously untreated subjects with non small cell lung cancer (NSCLC) or small cell lung cancer (SCLC). In: ClinicalTrials.gov [Internet]. Bethesda (MD): National Library of Medicine (US). 2000- [cited 2012 Feb 28]. Available from: http://clinicaltrials.gov/show/NCT00527735 NLM Identifier NCT00527735

Bristol-Myers Squibb. Trial in squamous non small cell lung cancer subjects comparing ipilimumab plus paclitaxel and carboplatin versus placebo plus paclitaxel and carboplatin. In: ClinicalTrials.gov [Internet]. Bethesda (MD): National Library of Medicine (US). 2000- [cited 2012 Feb 28]. Available from: http://clinicaltrials.gov/show/NCT01285609 NLM Identifier NCT01285609

Bugelski PJ, Achuthanandam R, Capocasale RJ, Treacy G, Bouman-Thio E. Monoclonal antibody-induced cytokine-release syndrome. *Expert Rev. Clin. Immunol.* 2009 sept;5(5):499–521.

Burger A, Heiss NS, Kreysch HG et al. The humanized monoclonal anti- EGFR antibody EMD 72000 potently inhibits the growth of EGFR-expressing human tumor xenografts insensitive to chemotherapeutic drugs [abstract 5719]. *Proc. Am. Assoc. Cancer Res.* 2003;44:1139.

Butts CA, Bodkin D, Middleman EL, Englund CW, Ellison D, Alam Y, et al. Randomized phase II study of gemcitabine plus cisplatin or carboplatin [corrected], with or without cetuximab, as first-line therapy for patients with advanced or metastatic non small-cell lung cancer. *J. Clin. Oncol.* 2007 déc 20;25(36):5777–84.

Byoung Chul Cho, Yonsei University. Phase II study of gefitinib plus nimotuzumab versus gefitinib in non-small cell lung cancer (DATE). In: ClinicalTrials.gov [Internet]. Bethesda (MD): National Library of Medicine (US). 2000- [cited 2012 Feb 28]. Available from: http://clinicaltrials.gov/show/NCT01498562 NLM Identifier: NCT01498562

Camacho LH. Novel therapies targeting the immune system: CTLA4 blockade with tremelimumab (CP-675,206), a fully human monoclonal antibody. *Expert Opin. Investig. Drugs.* 2008 mars;17(3):371–85.

Cappuzzo F, Varella-Garcia M, Shigematsu H, Domenichini I, Bartolini S, Ceresoli GL, et al. Increased HER2 gene copy number is associated with response to gefitinib therapy in epidermal growth factor receptor-positive non-small-cell lung cancer patients. *J. Clin. Oncol.* 2005 août 1;23(22):5007–18.

Carpenter G, Cohen S. Epidermal growth factor. *Annu. Rev. Biochem.* 1979;48:193–216.

Cartron G, Dacheux L, Salles G, Solal-Celigny P, Bardos P, Colombat P, et al. Therapeutic activity of humanized anti-CD20 monoclonal antibody and polymorphism in IgG Fc receptor FcgammaRIIIa gene. *Blood.* 2002 févr 1;99(3):754–8.

Cartron G, Trappe RU, Solal-Céligny P, Hallek M. Interindividual variability of response to rituximab: from biological origins to individualized therapies. *Clin. Cancer Res.* 2011 janv 1;17(1):19–30.

Cascone T, Morelli MP, Morgillo F, Kim W-Y, Rodolico G, Pepe S, et al. Synergistic anti-proliferative and pro-apoptotic activity of combined therapy with bortezomib, a proteasome inhibitor, with anti-epidermal growth factor receptor (EGFR) drugs in human cancer cells. *J. Cell. Physiol.* 2008 sept;216(3):698–707.

Clamon G, Herndon J, Kern J, Govindan R, Garst J, Watson D, et al. Lack of trastuzumab activity in nonsmall cell lung carcinoma with overexpression of erb-B2: 39810: a phase II trial of Cancer and Leukemia Group B. *Cancer.* 2005 avr 15;103(8):1670–5.

Clément-Duchêne C, Krupitskaya Y, Ganjoo K, Lavori P, McMillan A, Kumar A, et al. A phase II first-line study of gemcitabine, carboplatin, and bevacizumab in advanced stage nonsquamous non-small cell lung cancer. *J. Thorac. Oncol.* 2010 nov;5(11):1821–5.

Cohen BD, Baker DA, Soderstrom C, Tkalcevic G, Rossi AM, Miller PE, et al. Combination therapy enhances the inhibition of tumor growth with the fully human anti-type 1 insulin-like growth factor receptor monoclonal antibody CP-751,871. *Clin. Cancer Res.* 2005 mars 1;11(5):2063–73.

Cooper WA, Kohonen-Corish MRJ, Zhuang L, McCaughan B, Kennedy C, Screaton G, et al. Role and prognostic significance of tumor necrosis factor-related apoptosis-inducing ligand death receptor DR5 in nonsmall-cell lung cancer and precursor lesions. *Cancer.* 2008 juill 1;113(1):135–42.

Crinò L, Dansin E, Garrido P, Griesinger F, Laskin J, Pavlakis N, et al. Safety and efficacy of first-line bevacizumab-based therapy in advanced non-squamous non-small-cell lung cancer (SAiL, MO19390): a phase 4 study. *Lancet Oncol.* 2010 août;11(8):733–40.

Daleke DL. Regulation of transbilayer plasma membrane phospholipid asymmetry. *J. Lipid Res.* 2003 févr;44(2):233–42.

Dall'Acqua WF, Kiener PA, Wu H. Properties of human IgG1s engineered for enhanced binding to the neonatal Fc receptor (FcRn). *J. Biol. Chem.* 2006 août 18;281(33):23514–24.

Daydé D, Ternant D, Ohresser M, Lerondel S, Pesnel S, Watier H, et al. Tumor burden influences exposure and response to rituximab: pharmacokinetic-pharmacodynamic modeling using a syngeneic bioluminescent murine model expressing human CD20. *Blood.* 2009 avr 16;113(16):3765–72.

de Langen AJ, van den Boogaart V, Lubberink M, Backes WH, Marcus JT, van Tinteren H, et al. Monitoring response to antiangiogenic therapy in non-small cell lung cancer using imaging markers derived from PET and dynamic contrast-enhanced MRI. *J. Nucl. Med.* 2011 janv;52(1):48–55.

Descotes J. Immunotoxicity of monoclonal antibodies. MAbs. 2009 avr;1(2):104–11.

Digumarti R, Suresh AV, Bhattacharyya GS, Dasappa L, Shan J; Nizams Institute of Medical Sciences, Hyderabad, India; Yashoda Hospital, Hyderabad, India; Orchid Nursing Home, Kolkata, India; Kidwai Institute of Oncology, Bangalore, India; Peregrine Pharmaceuticals, Inc., Tustin, CA Phase II study of bavituximab plus paclitaxel and carboplatin in untreated locally advanced or metastatic non-small cell lung cancer: Interim results. *J. Clin. Oncol.* 2010;28 (15s), (suppl; abstr 7589)

Dingemans A-MC, de Langen AJ, van den Boogaart V, Marcus JT, Backes WH, Scholtens HTGM, et al. First-line erlotinib and bevacizumab in patients with locally advanced and/or metastatic non-small-cell lung cancer: a phase II study including molecular imaging. *Ann. Oncol.* 2011 mars;22(3):559–66.

Dowlati A, Gray R, Sandler AB, Schiller JH, Johnson DH. Cell adhesion molecules, vascular endothelial growth factor, and basic fibroblast growth factor in patients with non-small cell lung cancer treated with chemotherapy with or without bevacizumab--an Eastern Cooperative Oncology Group Study. *Clin. Cancer Res.* 2008 mars 1;14(5):1407–12.

Dudek AZ, Lesniewski-Kmak K, Shehadeh NJ, Pandey ON, Franklin M, Kratzke RA, et al. Phase I study of bortezomib and cetuximab in patients with solid tumours expressing epidermal growth factor receptor. *Br. J. Cancer.* 2009 mai 5;100(9):1379–84.

Ferrara N, Henzel WJ. Pituitary follicular cells secrete a novel heparin-binding growth factor specific for vascular endothelial cells. *Biochem. Biophys. Res. Commun.* 1989 juin 15;161(2):851–8.

Ferrara N. VEGF and the quest for tumour angiogenesis factors. *Nat. Rev. Cancer.* 2002 oct;2(10):795–803.

Ferrara N, Gerber H-P, LeCouter J. The biology of VEGF and its receptors. *Nat. Med.* 2003 juin;9(6):669–76.

Fontanini G, Boldrini L, Chinè S, Pisaturo F, Basolo F, Calcinai A, et al. Expression of vascular endothelial growth factor mRNA in non-small-cell lung carcinomas. *Br. J. Cancer.* 1999 janv;79(2):363–9.

Forero-Torres A, Shah J, Wood T, Posey J, Carlisle R, Copigneaux C, et al. Phase I trial of weekly tigatuzumab, an agonistic humanized monoclonal antibody targeting death receptor 5 (DR5). *Cancer Biother. Radiopharm.* 2010 févr;25(1):13–9.

Forero-Torres A, Shen S, Breitz H, Sims RB, Axworthy DB, Khazaeli MB, et al. Pretargeted radioimmunotherapy (RIT) with a novel anti-TAG-72 fusion protein. *Cancer Biother. Radiopharm.* 2005 août;20(4):379–90.

Franklin MC, Carey KD, Vajdos FF, Leahy DJ, de Vos AM, Sliwkowski MX. Insights into ErbB signaling from the structure of the ErbB2-pertuzumab complex. *Cancer Cell.* 2004 avr;5(4):317–28.

Freeman DJ, Bush T, Ogbagabriel S, Belmontes B, Juan T, Plewa C, et al. Activity of panitumumab alone or with chemotherapy in non-small cell lung carcinoma cell lines expressing mutant epidermal growth factor receptor. *Mol. Cancer Ther.* 2009 juin;8(6):1536–46.

Friess T, Scheuer W, Hasmann M. Combination treatment with erlotinib and pertuzumab against human tumor xenografts is superior to monotherapy. *Clin. Cancer Res.* 2005 juill 15;11(14):5300–9.

Fujio Y, Guo K, Mano T, Mitsuuchi Y, Testa JR, Walsh K. Cell cycle withdrawal promotes myogenic induction of Akt, a positive modulator of myocyte survival. *Mol. Cell. Biol.* 1999 juill;19(7):5073–82.

Fürstenberger G, Senn H-J. Insulin-like growth factors and cancer. *Lancet Oncol.* 2002 mai;3(5):298–302.

Galetta D, Pisconti S, Cinieri S, Pappagallo GL, Gebbia V, Borsellino N, et al. Induction pemetrexed and cisplatin followed by maintenance pemetrexed versus carboplatin plus paclitaxel plus bevacizumab followed by maintenance bevacizumab: a quality of life-oriented randomized phase III study in patients with advanced non-squamous non-small-cell lung cancer (ERACLE). *Clin Lung Cancer.* 2011 nov;12(6):402–6.

Gatzemeier U, Groth G, Butts C, Van Zandwijk N, Shepherd F, Ardizzoni A, et al. Randomized phase II trial of gemcitabine-cisplatin with or without trastuzumab in HER2-positive non-small-cell lung cancer. *Ann. Oncol.* 2004 janv;15(1):19–27.

Gatzemeier U, von Pawel J, Vynnychenko I, Zatloukal P, de Marinis F, Eberhardt WEE, et al. First-cycle rash and survival in patients with advanced non-small-cell lung cancer receiving cetuximab in combination with first-line chemotherapy: a subgroup analysis of data from the FLEX phase 3 study. *Lancet Oncol.* 2011 janv;12(1):30–7.

Gelderman KA, Tomlinson S, Ross GD, Gorter A. Complement function in mAb-mediated cancer immunotherapy. *Trends Immunol.* 2004 mars;25(3):158–64.

Gerber DE, Stopeck AT, Wong L, Rosen LS, Thorpe PE, Shan JS, et al. Phase I safety and pharmacokinetic study of bavituximab, a chimeric phosphatidylserine-targeting monoclonal antibody, in patients with advanced solid tumors. *Clin. Cancer Res.* 2011 nov 1;17(21):6888–96.

Gerber HP, McMurtrey A, Kowalski J, Yan M, Keyt BA, Dixit V, et al. Vascular endothelial growth factor regulates endothelial cell survival through the phosphatidylinositol 3'-kinase/Akt signal transduction pathway. Requirement for Flk-1/KDR activation. *J. Biol. Chem.* 1998 nov 13;273(46):30336–43.

Gesellschaft fur Medizinische Innovation – Hamatologie und Onkologie mbH. WiSP Wissenschaftlicher Service Pharma GmbH. Panitumumab plus pemetrexed and cisplatin (PemCisP) versus PemCis in the first-line treatment of patients with non-small cell lung cancer. In: ClinicalTrials.gov [Internet]. Bethesda (MD): National Library of Medicine (US). 2000- [cited 2012 Feb 28]. Available from: http://clinicaltrials.gov/show /NCT01088620 NLM Identifier NCT01088620

Getts DR, Getts MT, McCarthy DP, Chastain EML, Miller SD. Have we overestimated the benefit of human(ized) antibodies? *MAbs.* 2010 déc;2(6):682–94.

Goetsch L, Gonzalez A, Leger O, Beck A, Pauwels PJ, Haeuw JF, et al. A recombinant humanized anti-insulin-like growth factor receptor type I antibody (h7C10) enhances the antitumor activity of vinorelbine and anti-epidermal growth factor receptor therapy against human cancer xenografts. *Int. J. Cancer.* 2005 janv 10;113(2):316–28.

Goldenberg DM. Targeted therapy of cancer with radiolabeled antibodies. *J. Nucl. Med.* 2002 mai;43(5):693–713.

Gorski DH, Beckett MA, Jaskowiak NT, Calvin DP, Mauceri HJ, Salloum RM, et al. Blockage of the vascular endothelial growth factor stress response increases the antitumor effects of ionizing radiation. *Cancer Res.* 1999 juill 15;59(14):3374–8.

Govindan R, Bogart J, Stinchcombe T, Wang X, Hodgson L, Kratzke R, et al. Randomized phase II study of pemetrexed, carboplatin, and thoracic radiation with or without cetuximab in patients with locally advanced unresectable non-small-cell lung cancer: Cancer and Leukemia Group B trial 30407. *J. Clin. Oncol.* 2011 août 10;29(23):3120–5.

Greco FA, Bonomi P, Crawford J, Kelly K, Oh Y, Halpern W, et al. Phase 2 study of mapatumumab, a fully human agonistic monoclonal antibody which targets and activates the TRAIL receptor-1, in patients with advanced non-small cell lung cancer. *Lung Cancer.* 2008 juill;61(1):82–90.

Green MC, Murray JL, Hortobagyi GN. Monoclonal antibody therapy for solid tumors. *Cancer Treat. Rev.* 2000 août;26(4):269–86.

Gridelli C, Morabito A, Gebbia V, Mencoboni M, Carrozza F, Viganò MG, et al. Cetuximab and gemcitabine in elderly or adult PS2 patients with advanced non-small-cell lung cancer: The cetuximab in advanced lung cancer (CALC1-E and CALC1-PS2) randomized phase II trials. *Lung Cancer.* 2010 janv;67(1):86–92.

Gualberto A, Hixon ML, Karp DD, Li D, Green S, Dolled-Filhart M, et al. Pre-treatment levels of circulating free IGF-1 identify NSCLC patients who derive clinical benefit from figitumumab. *Br. J. Cancer.* 2011 janv 4;104(1):68–74.

Gualberto A. Figitumumab (CP-751,871) for cancer therapy. *Expert Opin. Biol. Ther.* 2010 avr;10(4):575–85.

Gualberto A, Dolled-Filhart MP, Hixon ML, et al. Molecular bases for sensitivity to figitumumab (CP-751,871) in NSCLC. *J. Clin. Oncol.* 2009; 27(15 suppl); Abstract 8091.

Gualberto A, Dolled-Filhart M, Gustavson M, Christiansen J, Wang Y-F, Hixon ML, et al. Molecular analysis of non-small cell lung cancer identifies subsets with different sensitivity to insulin-like growth factor I receptor inhibition. *Clin. Cancer Res.* 2010 sept 15;16(18):4654–65.

Gualberto A, Karp DD. Development of the monoclonal antibody figitumumab, targeting the insulin-like growth factor-1 receptor, for the treatment of patients with non-small-cell lung cancer. *Clin Lung Cancer.* 2009 juill;10(4):273–80.

Guarino MJ, Schneider CJ, Hosford MA, Brahmer JR, Rudin CM, Finckenstein FG, et al. Dual inhibition of the epidermal growth factor receptor pathway with cetuximab and erlotinib: a phase I study in patients with advanced solid malignancies. *Oncologist.* 2009 févr;14(2):119–24.

Hainsworth JD, Fang L, Huang JE, Karlin D, Russell K, Faoro L, et al. BRIDGE: an open-label phase II trial evaluating the safety of bevacizumab + carboplatin/paclitaxel as first-line treatment for patients with advanced, previously untreated, squamous non-small cell lung cancer. *J. Thorac. Oncol.* 2011 janv;6(1):109–14.

Hallqvist A, Wagenius G, Rylander H, Brodin O, Holmberg E, Lödén B, et al. Concurrent cetuximab and radiotherapy after docetaxel-cisplatin induction chemotherapy in stage III NSCLC: satellite--a phase II study from the Swedish Lung Cancer Study Group. *Lung Cancer.* 2011 févr;71(2):166–72.

Hanna N, Lilenbaum R, Ansari R, Lynch T, Govindan R, Jänne PA, et al. Phase II trial of cetuximab in patients with previously treated non-small-cell lung cancer. *J. Clin. Oncol.* 2006 nov 20;24(33):5253–8.

Hansel TT, Kropshofer H, Singer T, Mitchell JA, George AJT. The safety and side effects of monoclonal antibodies. *Nat. Rev. Drug Discov.* 2010 avr;9(4):325–38.

Hart TK, Cook RM, Zia-Amirhosseini P, Minthorn E, Sellers TS, Maleeff BE, et al. Preclinical efficacy and safety of mepolizumab (SB-240563), a humanized monoclonal antibody to IL-5, in cynomolgus monkeys. *J. Allergy Clin. Immunol.* 2001 août;108(2):250–7.

He J, Luster TA, Thorpe PE. Radiation-enhanced vascular targeting of human lung cancers in mice with a monoclonal antibody that binds anionic phospholipids. *Clin. Cancer Res.* 2007 sept 1;13(17):5211–8.

Heinmöller P, Gross C, Beyser K, Schmidtgen C, Maass G, Pedrocchi M, et al. HER2 status in non-small cell lung cancer: results from patient screening for enrollment to a phase II study of herceptin. *Clin. Cancer Res.* 2003 nov 1;9(14):5238–43.

Heist RS, Fidias P, Huberman M, Ardman B, Sequist LV, Temel JS, et al. A phase II study of oxaliplatin, pemetrexed, and bevacizumab in previously treated advanced non-small cell lung cancer. *J. Thorac. Oncol.* 2008 oct;3(10):1153–8.

Herbst RS, Ansari R, Bustin F, Flynn P, Hart L, Otterson GA, et al. Efficacy of bevacizumab plus erlotinib versus erlotinib alone in advanced non-small-cell lung cancer after failure of standard first-line chemotherapy (BeTa): a double-blind, placebo-controlled, phase 3 trial. *Lancet.* 2011 mai 28;377(9780):1846–54.

Herbst RS, Davies AM, Natale RB, Dang TP, Schiller JH, Garland LL, et al. Efficacy and safety of single-agent pertuzumab, a human epidermal receptor dimerization inhibitor, in patients with non small cell lung cancer. *Clin. Cancer Res.* 2007 oct 15;13(20):6175–81.

Herbst RS, Johnson DH, Mininberg E, Carbone DP, Henderson T, Kim ES, et al. Phase I/II trial evaluating the anti-vascular endothelial growth factor monoclonal antibody bevacizumab in combination with the HER-1/epidermal growth factor receptor tyrosine kinase inhibitor erlotinib for patients with recurrent non-small-cell lung cancer. *J. Clin. Oncol.* 2005 avr 10;23(11):2544–55.

Herbst RS, Kelly K, Chansky K, Mack PC, Franklin WA, Hirsch FR, et al. Phase II selection design trial of concurrent chemotherapy and cetuximab versus chemotherapy followed by cetuximab in advanced-stage non-small-cell lung cancer: Southwest Oncology Group study S0342. *J. Clin. Oncol.* 2010 nov 1;28(31):4747–54.

Herbst RS, Kurzrock R, Hong DS, Valdivieso M, Hsu C-P, Goyal L, et al. A first-in-human study of conatumumab in adult patients with advanced solid tumors. *Clin. Cancer Res.* 2010 déc 1;16(23):5883–91.

Herbst RS, O'Neill VJ, Fehrenbacher L, Belani CP, Bonomi PD, Hart L, et al. Phase II study of efficacy and safety of bevacizumab in combination with chemotherapy or erlotinib compared with chemotherapy alone for treatment of recurrent or refractory non small-cell lung cancer. *J. Clin. Oncol.* 2007 oct 20;25(30):4743–50.

Heymach JV, Nilsson M, Blumenschein G, Papadimitrakopoulou V, Herbst R. Epidermal growth factor receptor inhibitors in development for the treatment of non-small cell lung cancer. *Clin. Cancer Res.* 2006 juill 15;12(14 Pt 2):4441s–4445s.

Hirsch FR, Helfrich B, Franklin WA, Varella-Garcia M, Chan DC, Bunn PA Jr. Preclinical studies of gemcitabine and trastuzumab in breast and lung cancer cell lines. *Clin. Breast Cancer.* 2002 mai;3 Suppl 1:12–6.

Hirsch FR, Herbst RS, Olsen C, Chansky K, Crowley J, Kelly K, et al. Increased EGFR gene copy number detected by fluorescent in situ hybridization predicts outcome in non-small-cell lung cancer patients treated with cetuximab and chemotherapy. *J. Clin. Oncol.* 2008 juill 10;26(20):3351–7.

Hirsch FR, Herbst RS, Olsen C, Chansky K, Crowley J, Kelly K, et al. Increased EGFR gene copy number detected by fluorescent in situ hybridization predicts outcome in non-small-cell lung cancer patients treated with cetuximab and chemotherapy. *J. Clin. Oncol.* 2008 juill 10;26(20):3351–7.

Holtan SG, Creedon DJ. Mother knows best: lessons from fetomaternal tolerance applied to cancer immunity. *Front Biosci.* (Schol Ed). 2011;3:1533–40. http://www.ascopost.com/articles/november-2010/figitumumab-fails-to-improve-survival,-increases-toxicities,-in-first%E2%80%91line-treatment-of-patients-with-nsclc/

Hughes S, Liong J, Miah A, Ahmad S, Leslie M, Harper P, et al. A brief report on the safety study of induction chemotherapy followed by synchronous radiotherapy and cetuximab in stage III non-small cell lung cancer (NSCLC): SCRATCH study. *J. Thorac. Oncol.* 2008 juin;3(6):648–51.

Humblet Y. Cetuximab: an IgG(1) monoclonal antibody for the treatment of epidermal growth factor receptor-expressing tumours. *Expert Opin. Pharmacother.* 2004 juill;5(7):1621–33.

Hurwitz H, Fehrenbacher L, Novotny W, Cartwright T, Hainsworth J, Heim W, et al. Bevacizumab plus irinotecan, fluorouracil, and leucovorin for metastatic colorectal cancer. *N. Engl. J. Med.* 2004 juin 3;350(23):2335–42.

Hwang WYK, Foote J. Immunogenicity of engineered antibodies. *Methods.* 2005 mai;36(1):3–10.

Hynes NE, Lane HA. ERBB receptors and cancer: the complexity of targeted inhibitors. *Nat. Rev. Cancer.* 2005 mai;5(5):341–54.

Ichikawa K, Liu W, Zhao L, Wang Z, Liu D, Ohtsuka T, et al. Tumoricidal activity of a novel anti-human DR5 monoclonal antibody without hepatocyte cytotoxicity. *Nat. Med.* 2001 août;7(8):954–60.

ImClone LLC. A study of pemetrexed and carboplatin/cisplatin or gemcitabine and carboplatin/cisplatin with or without imc-1121b in patients previously untreated with recurrent or advanced non-small cell lung cancer (NSCLC). In: ClinicalTrials.gov [Internet]. Bethesda (MD): National Library of Medicine (US). 2000- [cited 2012 Feb

28]. Available from: http://clinicaltrials.gov/show/NCT01160744 NLM Identifier: NCT01160744.

ImClone LLC. A study of ramucirumab with paclitaxel and carboplatin in non-small cell lung cancer. In: ClinicalTrials.gov [Internet]. Bethesda (MD): National Library of Medicine (US). 2000- [cited 2012 Feb 28]. Available from: http://clinicaltrials.gov/show/NCT00735696 NLM Identifier: NCT00735696

ImClone LLC. Eli Lilly and Company. A study in second line non small cell lung cancer. In: ClinicalTrials.gov [Internet]. Bethesda (MD): National Library of Medicine (US). 2000- [cited 2012 Feb 28]. Available from: http://clinicaltrials.gov/show/NCT01168973 NLM Identifier: NCT01168973

ImClone LLC. A study of IMC-A12 (cixutumumab) with and without other standard chemotherapies in patients with lung cancer who have not received chemotherapy before. In: ClinicalTrials.gov [Internet]. Bethesda (MD): National Library of Medicine (US). 2000- [cited 2012 Feb 28]. Available from: http://clinicaltrials.gov/show/NCT00870870 NLM Identifier: NCT00870870

Inoue K, Slaton JW, Perrotte P, Davis DW, Bruns CJ, Hicklin DJ, et al. Paclitaxel enhances the effects of the anti-epidermal growth factor receptor monoclonal antibody ImClone C225 in mice with metastatic human bladder transitional cell carcinoma. *Clin. Cancer Res.* 2000 déc;6(12):4874–84.

Jalal S, Waterhouse D, Edelman MJ, Nattam S, Ansari R, Koneru K, et al. Pemetrexed plus cetuximab in patients with recurrent non-small cell lung cancer (NSCLC): a phase I/II study from the Hoosier Oncology Group. *J Thorac. Oncol.* 2009 nov;4(11):1420–4.

Jatoi A, Schild SE, Foster N, Henning GT, Dornfeld KJ, Flynn PJ, et al. A phase II study of cetuximab and radiation in elderly and/or poor performance status patients with locally advanced non-small-cell lung cancer (N0422). *Ann. Oncol.* 2010 oct;21(10):2040–4.

Jennewein M, Lewis MA, Zhao D, Tsyganov E, Slavine N, He J, et al. Vascular imaging of solid tumors in rats with a radioactive arsenic-labeled antibody that binds exposed phosphatidylserine. *Clin. Cancer Res.* 2008 mars 1;14(5):1377–85.

Jensen AD, Münter MW, Bischoff H, Haselmann R, Timke C, Krempien R, et al. Treatment of non-small cell lung cancer with intensity-modulated radiation therapy in combination with cetuximab: the NEAR protocol (NCT00115518). *BMC Cancer.* 2006;6:122.

Jensen AD, Münter MW, Bischoff HG, Haselmann R, Haberkorn U, Huber PE, et al. Combined treatment of nonsmall cell lung cancer NSCLC stage III with intensity-modulated RT radiotherapy and cetuximab: the NEAR trial. *Cancer.* 2011 juill 1;117(13):2986–94.

Johnson DH, Fehrenbacher L, Novotny WF, Herbst RS, Nemunaitis JJ, Jablons DM, et al. Randomized phase II trial comparing bevacizumab plus carboplatin and paclitaxel with carboplatin and paclitaxel alone in previously untreated locally advanced or metastatic non-small-cell lung cancer. *J. Clin. Oncol.* 2004 juin 1;22(11):2184–91.

Jones PT, Dear PH, Foote J, Neuberger MS, Winter G. Replacing the complementarity-determining regions in a human antibody with those from a mouse. *Nature.* 1986 juin 29;321(6069):522–5.

Jubb AM, Hurwitz HI, Bai W, Holmgren EB, Tobin P, Guerrero AS, et al. Impact of vascular endothelial growth factor-A expression, thrombospondin-2 expression, and microvessel density on the treatment effect of bevacizumab in metastatic colorectal cancer. *J. Clin. Oncol.* 2006 janv 10;24(2):217–27.

Kabbinavar FF, Wong JT, Ayala RE, et al The effect of antibody to vascular endothelial growth factor and cisplatin on the growth of lung tumors in nude mice[abstract]. *Proc. Am. Cancer Res.,* 36: 488 1995.

Kadota K, Huang C-L, Liu D, Ueno M, Kushida Y, Haba R, et al. The clinical significance of lymphangiogenesis and angiogenesis in non-small cell lung cancer patients. *Eur. J. Cancer.* 2008 mai;44(7):1057–67.

Kaneko E, Niwa R. Optimizing therapeutic antibody function: progress with Fc domain engineering. *BioDrugs.* 2011 févr 1;25(1):1–11.

Kaplan-Lefko PJ, Graves JD, Zoog SJ, Pan Y, Wall J, Branstetter DG, et al. Conatumumab, a fully human agonist antibody to death receptor 5, induces apoptosis via caspase activation in multiple tumor types. *Cancer Biol. Ther.* 2010 avr;9(8):618–31.

Karkkainen MJ, Mäkinen T, Alitalo K. Lymphatic endothelium: a new frontier of metastasis research. *Nat. Cell Biol.* 2002 janv;4(1):E2–5.

Karp DD, Paz-Ares LG, Novello S, Haluska P, Garland L, Cardenal F, et al. Phase II study of the anti-insulin-like growth factor type 1 receptor antibody CP-751,871 in combination with paclitaxel and carboplatin in previously untreated, locally advanced, or metastatic non-small-cell lung cancer. *J. Clin. Oncol.* 2009 mai 20;27(15):2516–22.

Karp DD, Pollak MN, Cohen RB, Eisenberg PD, Haluska P, Yin D, et al. Safety, pharmacokinetics, and pharmacodynamics of the insulin-like growth factor type 1 receptor inhibitor figitumumab (CP-751,871) in combination with paclitaxel and carboplatin. *J. Thorac. Oncol.* 2009 nov;4(11):1397–403.

Kawauchi K, Ogasawara T, Yasuyama M, Otsuka K, Yamada O. Regulation and importance of the PI3K/Akt/mTOR signaling pathway in hematologic malignancies. *Anticancer Agents Med. Chem.* 2009 nov;9(9):1024–38.

Keizer RJ, Huitema ADR, Schellens JHM, Beijnen JH. Clinical pharmacokinetics of therapeutic monoclonal antibodies. *Clin. Pharmacokinet.* 2010 août;49(8):493–507.

Khambata-Ford S, Harbison CT, Hart LL, Awad M, Xu L-A, Horak CE, et al. Analysis of potential predictive markers of cetuximab benefit in BMS099, a phase III study of cetuximab and first-line taxane/carboplatin in advanced non-small-cell lung cancer. *J. Clin. Oncol.* 2010 févr 20;28(6):918–27.

Kim ES, Mauer AM, William WN Jr, Tran HT, Liu D, Lee JJ, et al. A phase 2 study of cetuximab in combination with docetaxel in chemotherapy-refractory/resistant patients with advanced nonsmall cell lung cancer. *Cancer.* 2009 avr 15;115(8):1713–22.

Kim KJ, Li B, Winer J, Armanini M, Gillett N, Phillips HS, et al. Inhibition of vascular endothelial growth factor-induced angiogenesis suppresses tumour growth in vivo. *Nature.* 1993 avr 29;362(6423):841–4.

Kim SJ, Park Y, Hong HJ. Antibody engineering for the development of therapeutic antibodies. *Mol. Cells.* 2005 août 31;20(1):17–29.

Kim T. Technology evaluation: Matuzumab, Merck KGaA. *Curr. Opin. Mol. Ther.* 2004 févr;6(1):96–103.

Köhler G, Milstein C. Continuous cultures of fused cells secreting antibody of predefined specificity. *Nature.* 1975 août 7;256(5517):495–7.

Kollmannsberger C, Schittenhelm M, Honecker F, Tillner J, Weber D, Oechsle K, et al. A phase I study of the humanized monoclonal anti-epidermal growth factor receptor (EGFR) antibody EMD 72000 (matuzumab) in combination with paclitaxel in patients with EGFR-positive advanced non-small-cell lung cancer (NSCLC). *Ann. Oncol.* 2006 juin;17(6):1007–13.

Kollmannsberger C, Schittenhelm M, Honecker F, Tillner J, Weber D, Oechsle K, et al. A phase I study of the humanized monoclonal anti-epidermal growth factor receptor (EGFR) antibody EMD 72000 (matuzumab) in combination with paclitaxel in patients with EGFR-positive advanced non-small-cell lung cancer (NSCLC). *Ann. Oncol.* 2006 juin;17(6):1007–13.

Kozin SV, Boucher Y, Hicklin DJ, Bohlen P, Jain RK, Suit HD. Vascular endothelial growth factor receptor-2-blocking antibody potentiates radiation-induced long-term control of human tumor xenografts. *Cancer Res.* 2001 janv 1;61(1):39–44.

Kuenen B, Witteveen PO, Ruijter R, Giaccone G, Dontabhaktuni A, Fox F, et al. A phase I pharmacologic study of necitumumab (IMC-11F8), a fully human IgG1 monoclonal antibody directed against EGFR in patients with advanced solid malignancies. *Clin. Cancer Res.* 2010 mars 15;16(6):1915–23.

Kuo TT, Baker K, Yoshida M, Qiao S-W, Aveson VG, Lencer WI, et al. Neonatal Fc Receptor: From Immunity to Therapeutics. *J. Clin. Immunol.* 2010 nov;30(6):777–89.

Lara PN Jr, Laptalo L, Longmate J, Lau DHM, Gandour-Edwards R, Gumerlock PH, et al. Trastuzumab plus docetaxel in HER2/neu-positive non-small-cell lung cancer: a California Cancer Consortium screening and phase II trial. *Clin. Lung Cancer.* 2004 janv;5(4):231–6.

Laskin J, Crinò L, Felip E, Franke F, Gorbunova V, Groen H, et al. Safety and efficacy of first-line bevacizumab plus chemotherapy in elderly patients with advanced or recurrent nonsquamous non-small cell lung cancer: safety of avastin in lung trial (MO19390). *J. Thorac. Oncol.* 2012 janv;7(1):203–11.

Lee CG, Heijn M, di Tomaso E, Griffon-Etienne G, Ancukiewicz M, Koike C, et al. Anti-Vascular endothelial growth factor treatment augments tumor radiation response under normoxic or hypoxic conditions. *Cancer Res.* 2000 oct 1;60(19):5565–70.

Leighl NB, Zatloukal P, Mezger J, Ramlau R, Moore N, Reck M, et al. Efficacy and safety of bevacizumab-based therapy in elderly patients with advanced or recurrent nonsquamous non-small cell lung cancer in the phase III BO17704 study (AVAiL). *J. Thorac. Oncol.* 2010 déc;5(12):1970–6.

Lewis, W. H. The vascular pattern of tumors. *Johns Hopkins Hosp. Bull.* 41, 156–162 (1927).

Lilenbaum R, Raez L, Tseng J, Seigel L, Davila E. Efficacy and safety of oxaliplatin and gemcitabine with bevacizumab in advanced non-small cell lung cancer. *J. Thorac. Oncol.* 2008 mai;3(5):511–5.

Linke R, Klein A, Seimetz D. Catumaxomab: clinical development and future directions. *MAbs.* 2010 avr;2(2):129–36.

Lu J-F, Bruno R, Eppler S, Novotny W, Lum B, Gaudreault J. Clinical pharmacokinetics of bevacizumab in patients with solid tumors. *Cancer Chemother. Pharmacol.* 2008 oct;62(5):779–86.

Luster TA, Carrell JA, McCormick K, Sun D, Humphreys R. Mapatumumab and lexatumumab induce apoptosis in TRAIL-R1 and TRAIL-R2 antibody-resistant NSCLC cell lines when treated in combination with bortezomib. *Mol. Cancer Ther.* 2009 févr;8(2):292–302.

Luster TA, Carrell JA, McCormick K, Sun D, Humphreys R. Mapatumumab and lexatumumab induce apoptosis in TRAIL-R1 and TRAIL-R2 antibody-resistant NSCLC cell lines when treated in combination with bortezomib. *Mol. Cancer Ther.* 2009 févr;8(2):292–302.

Lynch TJ, Patel T, Dreisbach L, McCleod M, Heim WJ, Hermann RC, et al. Cetuximab and first-line taxane/carboplatin chemotherapy in advanced non-small-cell lung cancer: results of the randomized multicenter phase III trial BMS099. *J. Clin. Oncol.* 2010 févr 20;28(6):911–7.

Maemondo M, Inoue A, Kobayashi K, Sugawara S, Oizumi S, Isobe H, et al. Gefitinib or chemotherapy for non-small-cell lung cancer with mutated EGFR. *N. Engl. J. Med.* 2010 juin 24;362(25):2380–8.

Maillet A, Congy-Jolivet N, Le Guellec S, Vecellio L, Hamard S, Courty Y, et al. Aerodynamical, immunological and pharmacological properties of the anticancer antibody cetuximab following nebulization. *Pharm. Res.* 2008 juin;25(6):1318–26.

Maillet A, Guilleminault L, Lemarié E, Lerondel S, Azzopardi N, Montharu J, et al. The airways, a novel route for delivering monoclonal antibodies to treat lung tumors. *Pharm. Res.* 2011 sept;28(9):2147–56.

Malykh YN, Schauer R, Shaw L. N-Glycolylneuraminic acid in human tumours. *Biochimie.* 2001 juill;83(7):623–34.

Mantovani A, Allavena P, Sica A, Balkwill F. Cancer-related inflammation. *Nature.* 2008 juill 24;454(7203):436–44.

Marini P. Drug evaluation: lexatumumab, an intravenous human agonistic mAb targeting TRAIL receptor 2. *Curr. Opin. Mol. Ther.* 2006 déc;8(6):539–46.

Matar P, Rojo F, Cassia R, Moreno-Bueno G, Di Cosimo S, Tabernero J, et al. Combined epidermal growth factor receptor targeting with the tyrosine kinase inhibitor gefitinib (ZD1839) and the monoclonal antibody cetuximab (IMC-C225): superiority over single-agent receptor targeting. *Clin. Cancer Res.* 2004 oct 1;10(19):6487–501.

Mateo C, Moreno E, Amour K, Lombardero J, Harris W, Pérez R. Humanization of a mouse monoclonal antibody that blocks the epidermal growth factor receptor: recovery of antagonistic activity. *Immunotechnology.* 1997 mars;3(1):71–81.

Mendel DB, Laird AD, Xin X, Louie SG, Christensen JG, Li G, et al. In vivo antitumor activity of SU11248, a novel tyrosine kinase inhibitor targeting vascular endothelial growth factor and platelet-derived growth factor receptors: determination of a pharmacokinetic/pharmacodynamic relationship. *Clin. Cancer Res.* 2003 janv;9(1):327–37.

Merck. A study evaluating dalotuzumab (MK0646) in combination with erlotinib for patients with non-small cell lung cancer (0646-007). In: ClinicalTrials.gov [Internet]. Bethesda (MD): National Library of Medicine (US). 2000- [cited 2012 Feb 28]. Available from: http://clinicaltrials.gov/show/NCT00654420 NLM Identifier: NCT00654420

Merck. University of Kansas. MK-0646 insulin growth factor 1 receptor antibody in stage IIIb or IV metastatic non-squamous lung cancer (IMPACT). In: ClinicalTrials.gov [Internet]. Bethesda (MD): National Library of Medicine (US). 2000- [cited 2012 Feb 28]. Available from: http://clinicaltrials.gov/show/NCT00799240 NLM Identifier: NCT00799240

Miller VA, O'Connor P, Soh C, Kabbinavar F. A randomized, double-blind, placebo-controlled, phase IIIb trial (ATLAS) comparing bevacizumab (B) therapy with or without erlotinib (E) after completion of chemotherapy with B for first-line treatment of locally advanced, recurrent, or metastatic non-small cell lung cancer (NSCLC). *J. Clin. Oncol.* 2009;27(Suppl.):8002.

Molife LR, Fong PC, Paccagnella L, Reid AHM, Shaw HM, Vidal L, et al. The insulin-like growth factor-I receptor inhibitor figitumumab (CP-751,871) in combination with docetaxel in patients with advanced solid tumours: results of a phase Ib dose-escalation, open-label study. *Br. J. Cancer.* 2010 juill 27;103(3):332–9.

Nakagawa M, Uramoto H, Oka S, Chikaishi Y, Iwanami T, Shimokawa H, et al. Clinical Significance of IGF1R Expression in Non-Small-Cell Lung Cancer. *Clin. Lung Cancer.* 2012 mars;13(2):136–42.

National Cancer Institute (NCI). North Central Cancer Treatment Group. Cancer and leukemia group b. high-dose or standard-dose radiation therapy and chemotherapy with or without cetuximab in treating patients with newly diagnosed stage iii non-small cell lung cancer that cannot be removed by surgery. In: ClinicalTrials.gov [Internet]. Bethesda (MD): National Library of Medicine (US). 2000- [cited 2012 Feb 28]. Available from: http://clinicaltrials.gov/show/NCT00533949 NLM Identifier: NCT00533949

National Cancer Institute (NCI), Chemotherapy and radiation therapy with or without panitumumab in treating patients with stage IIIA non-small cell lung cancer. In: ClinicalTrials.gov [Internet]. Bethesda (MD): National Library of Medicine (US). 2000- [cited 2012 Feb 28]. Available from: http://clinicaltrials.gov/show/NCT00979212 NLM Identifier NCT00979212

National Cancer Institute (NCI). Gemcitabine hydrochloride and carboplatin with or without MK-0646 as first-line therapy in treating patients with stage IIIB or Stage IV non-small cell lung cancer. In: ClinicalTrials.gov [Internet]. Bethesda (MD): National Library of Medicine (US). 2000- [cited 2012 Feb 28]. Available from: http://clinicaltrials.gov/show /NCT00951444 NLM Identifier: NCT00951444

National Cancer Institute (NCI). Paclitaxel, Carboplatin, and bevacizumab with or without cixutumumab in treating patients with stage IV or recurrent non-small cell lung cancer. In: ClinicalTrials.gov [Internet]. Bethesda (MD): National Library of Medicine (US). 2000- [cited 2012 Feb 28]. Available from: http://clinicaltrials.gov/show/NCT00955305 NLM Identifier: NCT00955305

National Cancer Institute (NCI). Erlotinib with or without IMC-A12 in treating patients with stage III or Stage IV non-small cell lung cancer. In: ClinicalTrials.gov [Internet]. Bethesda (MD): National Library of Medicine (US). 2000- [cited 2012 Feb 28]. Available from: http://clinicaltrials.gov/show/NCT00778167 NLM Identifier: NCT00778167

Neal JW, Heist RS, Fidias P, Temel JS, Huberman M, Marcoux JP, et al. Cetuximab monotherapy in patients with advanced non-small cell lung cancer after prior epidermal growth factor receptor tyrosine kinase inhibitor therapy. *J. Thorac. Oncol.* 2010 nov;5(11):1855–8.

Nezlin R. Interactions between immunoglobulin G molecules. *Immunol. Lett.* 2010 août 16;132(1-2):1–5.

Nishinaka T, Yabe-Nishimura C. EGF receptor-ERK pathway is the major signaling pathway that mediates upregulation of aldose reductase expression under oxidative stress. *Free Radic. Biol. Med.* 2001 juill 15;31(2):205–16.

Nissim A, Chernajovsky Y. Historical development of monoclonal antibody therapeutics. *Handb. Exp. Pharmacol.* 2008;(181):3–18.

Nuijten M, Heigener DF, Bischoff HG, Chouaid C, Vergnenègre A, de Castro Carpeño J, et al. Effectiveness of bevacizumab- and pemetrexed-cisplatin treatment for patients with advanced non-squamous non-small cell lung cancer. *Lung Cancer.* 2010 août;69 Suppl 1:S4–10.

O'Farrell A-M, Abrams TJ, Yuen HA, Ngai TJ, Louie SG, Yee KWH, et al. SU11248 is a novel FLT3 tyrosine kinase inhibitor with potent activity in vitro and in vivo. *Blood.* 2003 mai 1;101(9):3597–605.

Oliva JL, Griner EM, Kazanietz MG. PKC isozymes and diacylglycerol-regulated proteins as effectors of growth factor receptors. *Growth Factors.* 2005 déc;23(4):245–52.

Olofsson B, Jeltsch M, Eriksson U, Alitalo K. Current biology of VEGF-B and VEGF-C. *Curr. Opin. Biotechnol.* 1999 déc;10(6):528–35.

Paintaud G. [Pharmacokinetics (PK) of mAbs]. *Med. Sci.* (Paris). 2009 déc;25(12):1057–62.

Parexel. PPD Medidata Solutions. Laboratory Corporation of America. University of Colorado, Denver. Thermo Fisher Scientific. ImClone LLC. First-line treatment of patients with stage iv nonsquamous non-small cell lung cancer with necitumumab (IMC-11F8) and pemetrexed-cisplatin (INSPIRE). In: ClinicalTrials.gov [Internet]. Bethesda (MD): National Library of Medicine (US). 2000- [cited 2012 Feb 28]. Available from: http://clinicaltrials.gov/show/NCT00982111 NLM Identifier: NCT00982111

Pasche N, Neri D. Immunocytokines: a novel class of potent armed antibodies. Drug Discovery Today [Internet]. 2012 janv 24 [cité 2012 mars 1]; Available de: http://www.ncbi.nlm.nih.gov/pubmed/22289353

Patel JD, Bonomi P, Socinski MA, Govindan R, Hong S, Obasaju C, et al. Treatment rationale and study design for the pointbreak study: a randomized, open-label phase III study of pemetrexed/carboplatin/bevacizumab followed by maintenance pemetrexed/bevacizumab versus paclitaxel/carboplatin/bevacizumab followed by maintenance bevacizumab in patients with stage IIIB or IV nonsquamous non-small-cell lung cancer. *Clin. Lung Cancer.* 2009 juill;10(4):252–6.

Patel JD, Hensing TA, Rademaker A, Hart EM, Blum MG, Milton DT, et al. Phase II study of pemetrexed and carboplatin plus bevacizumab with maintenance pemetrexed and bevacizumab as first-line therapy for nonsquamous non-small-cell lung cancer. *J. Clin. Oncol.* 2009 juill 10;27(20):3284–9.

Patel RD, Momi RS, Hariprasad SM. Review of ranibizumab trials for neovascular age-related macular degeneration. *Semin. Ophthalmol.* 2011 nov;26(6):372–9.

Paudyal P, Paudyal B, Hanaoka H, Oriuchi N, Iida Y, Yoshioka H, et al. Imaging and biodistribution of Her2/neu expression in non-small cell lung cancer xenografts with Cu-labeled trastuzumab PET. *Cancer Sci.* 2010 avr;101(4):1045–50.

Peregrine Pharmaceuticals. Study of paclitaxel/carboplatin with or without bavituximab in previously untreated non small-cell lung cancer. In: ClinicalTrials.gov [Internet]. Bethesda (MD): National Library of Medicine (US). 2000- [cited 2012 Feb 28]. Available from: http://clinicaltrials.gov/show/NCT01160601 NLM Identifier NCT01160601

Peregrine Pharmaceuticals. Study of Bavituximab Plus Docetaxel in Patients With Locally Advanced or Metastatic Non-Squamous Non Small-Cell Lung Cancer. In: ClinicalTrials.gov [Internet]. Bethesda (MD): National Library of Medicine (US). 2000-

[cited 2012 Feb 28]. Available from: http://clinicaltrials.gov/show/NCT01138163 NLM Identifier NCT01138163

Pfizer. Carboplatin and paclitaxel with or without CP-751, 871 (an IGF-1R inhibitor) for advanced NSCLC of squamous, large cell and adenosquamous carcinoma histology. In: ClinicalTrials.gov [Internet]. Bethesda (MD): National Library of Medicine (US). 2000- [cited 2012 Feb 28]. Available from: http://clinicaltrials.gov/show/NCT00596830 NLM Identifier: NCT00596830

Pfizer. Trial of CP-751, 871 and erlotinib in refractory lung cancer (NSCLC). In: ClinicalTrials.gov [Internet]. Bethesda (MD): National Library of Medicine (US). 2000- [cited 2012 Feb 28]. Available from: http://clinicaltrials.gov/show/NCT00673049 NLM Identifier: NCT00673049

Pfizer. Randomized study of CP-675,206 or best supportive care immediately after platinum-based therapy for non-small cell lung cancer (NSCLC). . In: ClinicalTrials.gov [Internet]. Bethesda (MD): National Library of Medicine (US). 2000- [cited 2012 Feb 28]. Available from: http://clinicaltrials.gov/show/NCT00312975 NLM Identifier NCT00312975

Pham CD, Roberts TP, van Bruggen N, Melnyk O, Mann J, Ferrara N, et al. Magnetic resonance imaging detects suppression of tumor vascular permeability after administration of antibody to vascular endothelial growth factor. *Cancer Invest.* 1998;16(4):225–30.

Piccart-Gebhart MJ, Procter M, Leyland-Jones B, Goldhirsch A, Untch M, Smith I, et al. Trastuzumab after adjuvant chemotherapy in HER2-positive breast cancer. *N. Engl. J. Med.* 2005 oct 20;353(16):1659–72.

Pirker R, Pereira JR, Szczesna A, von Pawel J, Krzakowski M, Ramlau R, et al. Cetuximab plus chemotherapy in patients with advanced non-small-cell lung cancer (FLEX): an open-label randomised phase III trial. *Lancet.* 2009 mai 2;373(9674):1525–31.

Pirker R, Pereira JR, von Pawel J, Krzakowski M, Ramlau R, Park K, et al. EGFR expression as a predictor of survival for first-line chemotherapy plus cetuximab in patients with advanced non-small-cell lung cancer: analysis of data from the phase 3 FLEX study. *Lancet Oncol.* 2012 janv;13(1):33–42.

Pouget J-P, Navarro-Teulon I, Bardiès M, Chouin N, Cartron G, Pèlegrin A, et al. Clinical radioimmunotherapy--the role of radiobiology. *Nat. Rev. Clin. Oncol.* 2011;8(12):720–34.

Press Release: Lilly. Bristol-Myers Squibb Stop Enrollment in One of Two Phase III Lung Cancer Trials of Necitumumab. Princeton, NJ: Bristol-Myers Squibb, 2011.Available from: http://www.bms.com/news/press_releases/pages/default.aspx?RSSLink=http://www.businesswire.com/news/bms/20110202006011/enandt=634322838509124725)

Presta LG, Chen H, O'Connor SJ, Chisholm V, Meng YG, Krummen L, et al. Humanization of an anti-vascular endothelial growth factor monoclonal antibody for the therapy of solid tumors and other disorders. *Cancer Res.* 1997 oct 15;57(20):4593–9.

Prewett M, Bassi R, Youssoufian H, et al. The fully human EGFR antibody IMC-11F8 significantly increases the antitumor effects of cisplatin plus gemcitabine in human non-small cell lung cancer models. *Proc. Am. Assoc. Cancer Res.* 2009;abstract 2774.

Pukac L, Kanakaraj P, Humphreys R, Alderson R, Bloom M, Sung C, et al. HGS-ETR1, a fully human TRAIL-receptor 1 monoclonal antibody, induces cell death in multiple tumour types in vitro and in vivo. *Br. J. Cancer.* 2005 avr 25;92(8):1430–41.

Raben D, Helfrich B, Chan DC, Ciardiello F, Zhao L, Franklin W, et al. The effects of cetuximab alone and in combination with radiation and/or chemotherapy in lung cancer. *Clin. Cancer Res.* 2005 janv 15;11(2 Pt 1):795–805.

Rajkumar SV, Richardson PG, Hideshima T, Anderson KC. Proteasome inhibition as a novel therapeutic target in human cancer. *J. Clin. Oncol.* 2005 janv 20;23(3):630–9.

Ramalingam S, Forster J, Naret C, Evans T, Sulecki M, Lu H, et al. Dual inhibition of the epidermal growth factor receptor with cetuximab, an IgG1 monoclonal antibody, and gefitinib, a tyrosine kinase inhibitor, in patients with refractory non-small cell lung cancer (NSCLC): a phase I study. *J. Thorac. Oncol.* 2008 mars;3(3):258–64.

Ramalingam SS, Dahlberg SE, Langer CJ, Gray R, Belani CP, Brahmer JR, et al. Outcomes for elderly, advanced-stage non small-cell lung cancer patients treated with bevacizumab in combination with carboplatin and paclitaxel: analysis of Eastern Cooperative Oncology Group Trial 4599. *J. Clin. Oncol.* 2008 janv 1;26(1):60–5.

Ramalingam SS, Lee J-W, Belani CP, Aisner SC, Kolesar J, Howe C, et al. Cetuximab for the treatment of advanced bronchioloalveolar carcinoma (BAC): an Eastern Cooperative Oncology Group phase II study (ECOG 1504). *J. Clin. Oncol.* 2011 mai 1;29(13):1709–14.

Ramalingam SS, Spigel DR, Chen D, Steins MB, Engelman JA, Schneider C-P, et al. Randomized phase II study of erlotinib in combination with placebo or R1507, a monoclonal antibody to insulin-like growth factor-1 receptor, for advanced-stage non-small-cell lung cancer. *J. Clin. Oncol.* 2011 déc 1;29(34):4574–80.

Rasul KI, Kerr DJ. Targeted therapies: Cetuximab plus chemotherapy in patients with advanced NSCLC. *Nat. Rev. Clin. Oncol.* 2009 sept;6(9):499–500.

Reck M, von Pawel J, Zatloukal P, Ramlau R, Gorbounova V, Hirsh V, et al. Phase III trial of cisplatin plus gemcitabine with either placebo or bevacizumab as first-line therapy for nonsquamous non-small-cell lung cancer: AVAil. *J. Clin. Oncol.* 2009 mars 10;27(8):1227–34.

Rigas JR, Schuster M, Orlov SV, et al. Effect of ALD518, a humanized anti-IL-6 antibody, on lean body mass loss and symptoms in patients with advanced non-small cell lung cancer (NSCLC): results of a phase II randomized, double-blind safety and efficacy trial. *J. Clin. Oncol.* 2010;28(15s):abstract 7622 33.

Reichert JM. Which are the antibodies to watch in 2012? *MAbs.* 2012 janv 1;4(1):1–3.

Robert F, Blumenschein G, Herbst RS, Fossella FV, Tseng J, Saleh MN, et al. Phase I/IIa study of cetuximab with gemcitabine plus carboplatin in patients with chemotherapy-naive advanced non-small-cell lung cancer. *J. Clin. Oncol.* 2005 déc 20;23(36):9089–96.

Robert F, Busby EM, LoBuglio AF. Chemotherapy tolerance after radioimmunotherapy with 90Y-CC49 monoclonal antibody in patients with advanced non-small cell lung cancer: clinical effects and hematologic toxicity. *Cancer Biother. Radiopharm.* 2003 juin;18(3):317–25.

Roche Pharma AG. Genentech. A study of the combination of erlotinib and pertuzumab in patients with relapsed non-small cell lung cancer (PENGUIN). In: ClinicalTrials.gov [Internet]. Bethesda (MD): National Library of Medicine (US). 2000- [cited 2012 Feb 28]. Available from: http://clinicaltrials.gov/show/NCT00855894 NLM Identifier: NCT00855894

Rojas R, Apodaca G. Immunoglobulin transport across polarized epithelial cells. *Nat. Rev. Mol. Cell Biol.* 2002 déc;3(12):944–55.

Rosell R, Robinet G, Szczesna A, Ramlau R, Constenla M, Mennecier BC, et al. Randomized phase II study of cetuximab plus cisplatin/vinorelbine compared with cisplatin/vinorelbine alone as first-line therapy in EGFR-expressing advanced non-small-cell lung cancer. *Ann. Oncol.* 2008 févr;19(2):362–9.

Roskoski R Jr. Vascular endothelial growth factor (VEGF) signaling in tumor progression. *Crit. Rev. Oncol. Hematol.* 2007 juin;62(3):179–213.

Ross HJ, Hart LL, Swanson PM, Rarick MU, Figlin RA, Jacobs AD, et al. A randomized, multicenter study to determine the safety and efficacy of the immunoconjugate SGN-15 plus docetaxel for the treatment of non-small cell lung carcinoma. *Lung Cancer.* 2006 oct;54(1):69–77.

Ross JS, Gray K, Gray GS, Worland PJ, Rolfe M. Anticancer antibodies. *Am. J. Clin. Pathol.* 2003 avr;119(4):472–85.

Rudnick SI, Lou J, Shaller CC, Tang Y, Klein-Szanto AJP, Weiner LM, et al. Influence of affinity and antigen internalization on the uptake and penetration of Anti-HER2 antibodies in solid tumors. *Cancer Res.* 2011 mars 15;71(6):2250–9.

Rusch V, Klimstra D, Venkatraman E, Pisters PW, Langenfeld J, Dmitrovsky E. Overexpression of the epidermal growth factor receptor and its ligand transforming growth factor alpha is frequent in resectable non-small cell lung cancer but does not predict tumor progression. *Clin. Cancer Res.* 1997 avr;3(4):515–22.

Sabel MS, Hess SD, Egilmez NK, Conway TF Jr, Chen F-A, Bankert RB. CTLA-4 blockade augments human T lymphocyte-mediated suppression of lung tumor xenografts in SCID mice. *Cancer Immunol. Immunother.* 2005 oct;54(10):944–52.

Sakai K, Yokote H, Murakami-Murofushi K, Tamura T, Saijo N, Nishio K. Pertuzumab, a novel HER dimerization inhibitor, inhibits the growth of human lung cancer cells mediated by the HER3 signaling pathway. *Cancer Sci.* 2007 sept;98(9):1498–503.

Sandler A, Gray R, Perry MC, Brahmer J, Schiller JH, Dowlati A, et al. Paclitaxel-carboplatin alone or with bevacizumab for non-small-cell lung cancer. *N. Engl. J. Med.* 2006 déc 14;355(24):2542–50.

Sandomenico C, Costanzo R, Carillio G, Piccirillo MC, Montanino A, Di Maio M, et al. Bevacizumab in Non Small Cell Lung Cancer: Development, Current Status and Issues. Current Medicinal Chemistry [Internet]. 2012 janv 2 [cité 2012 mars 1]; Available de: http://www.ncbi.nlm.nih.gov/pubmed/22214464

Scagliotti GV, Novello S. The role of the insulin-like growth factor signaling pathway in non-small cell lung cancer and other solid tumors. Cancer Treat. Rev. [Internet]. 2011 sept 8 [cité 2012 mars 1]; Available de: http://www.ncbi.nlm.nih.gov/pubmed/21907495

Scagliotti GV, Parikh P, von Pawel J, Biesma B, Vansteenkiste J, Manegold C, et al. Phase III study comparing cisplatin plus gemcitabine with cisplatin plus pemetrexed in chemotherapy-naive patients with advanced-stage non-small-cell lung cancer. *J. Clin. Oncol.* 2008 juill 20;26(21):3543–51.

Scheuer W, Friess T, Burtscher H, Bossenmaier B, Endl J, Hasmann M. Strongly enhanced antitumor activity of trastuzumab and pertuzumab combination treatment on HER2-positive human xenograft tumor models. *Cancer Res.* 2009 déc 15;69(24):9330–6.

Schiller JH, von Pawel J, Schütt P, Ansari RH, Thomas M, Saleh M, et al. Pemetrexed with or without matuzumab as second-line treatment for patients with stage IIIB/IV non-small cell lung cancer. *J. Thorac. Oncol.* 2010 déc;5(12):1977–85.

Schittenhelm MM, Kollmannsberger C, Oechsle K, Harlow A, Morich J, Honecker F, et al. Molecular determinants of response to matuzumab in combination with paclitaxel for patients with advanced non-small cell lung cancer. *Mol. Cancer Ther.* 2009 mars;8(3):481–9.

Schuster M, Rigas JR, Orlov SV, et al. ALD518, a humanized anti-IL-6 antibody, treats anemia in patients with advanced non-small cell lung cancer (NSCLC): results of a phase II, randomized, double-blind, placebo-controlled trial. *J. Clin. Oncol.* 2010;28(15s):abstract 7631.

Sebastian M, Passlick B, Friccius-Quecke H, Jäger M, Lindhofer H, Kanniess F, et al. Treatment of non-small cell lung cancer patients with the trifunctional monoclonal antibody catumaxomab (anti-EpCAM x anti-CD3): a phase I study. *Cancer Immunol. Immunother.* 2007 oct;56(10):1637–44.

Sebolt-Leopold JS. MEK inhibitors: a therapeutic approach to targeting the Ras-MAP kinase pathway in tumors. *Curr. Pharm. Des.* 2004;10(16):1907–14.

Shawler DL, Bartholomew RM, Smith LM, Dillman RO. Human immune response to multiple injections of murine monoclonal IgG. *J. Immunol.* 1985 août;135(2):1530–5.

Shepherd FA, Rodrigues Pereira J, Ciuleanu T, Tan EH, Hirsh V, Thongprasert S, et al. Erlotinib in previously treated non-small-cell lung cancer. *N. Engl. J. Med.* 2005 juill 14;353(2):123–32.

Shepherd FA, Rodrigues Pereira J, Ciuleanu T, Tan EH, Hirsh V, Thongprasert S, et al. Erlotinib in previously treated non-small-cell lung cancer. *N. Engl. J. Med.* 2005 juill 14;353(2):123–32.

Shimada O, Wu X, Jin X, Nouh MAA-M, Fiscella M, Albert V, et al. Human agonistic antibody to tumor necrosis factor-related apoptosis-inducing ligand receptor 2 induces cytotoxicity and apoptosis in prostate cancer and bladder cancer cells. *Urology.* 2007 févr;69(2):395–401.

Slamon DJ, Leyland-Jones B, Shak S, Fuchs H, Paton V, Bajamonde A, et al. Use of chemotherapy plus a monoclonal antibody against HER2 for metastatic breast cancer that overexpresses HER2. *N. Engl. J. Med.* 2001 mars 15;344(11):783–92.

Socinski MA, Saleh MN, Trent DF, Dobbs TW, Zehngebot LM, Levine MA, et al. A randomized, phase II trial of two dose schedules of carboplatin/paclitaxel/cetuximab in stage IIIB/IV non-small-cell lung cancer (NSCLC). *Ann. Oncol.* 2009 juin;20(6):1068–73.

Socinski MA. Antibodies to the epidermal growth factor receptor in non small cell lung cancer: current status of matuzumab and panitumumab. *Clin. Cancer Res.* 2007 août 1;13(15 Pt 2):s4597–4601.

Socinski MA, Scappaticci FA, Samant M, Kolb MM, Kozloff MF. Safety and efficacy of combining sunitinib with bevacizumab + paclitaxel/carboplatin in non-small cell lung cancer. *J. Thorac. Oncol.* 2010 mars;5(3):354–60.

Songür N, Kuru B, Kalkan F, Ozdilekcan C, Cakmak H, Hizel N. Serum interleukin-6 levels correlate with malnutrition and survival in patients with advanced non-small cell lung cancer. *Tumori.* 2004 avr;90(2):196–200.

Spierings DCJ, de Vries EGE, Timens W, Groen HJM, Boezen HM, de Jong S. Expression of TRAIL and TRAIL death receptors in stage III non-small cell lung cancer tumors. *Clin. Cancer Res.* 2003 août 15;9(9):3397–405.

Spigel DR, Greco FA, Thompson DS, Webb C, Rubinsak J, Inhorn RC, et al. Phase II study of cetuximab, docetaxel, and gemcitabine in patients with previously untreated advanced non-small-cell lung cancer. *Clin. Lung Cancer.* 2010 mai;11(3):198–203.

Spigel DR, Greco FA, Zubkus JD, Murphy PB, Saez RA, Farley C, et al. Phase II trial of irinotecan, carboplatin, and bevacizumab in the treatment of patients with extensive-stage small-cell lung cancer. *J. Thorac. Oncol.* 2009 déc;4(12):1555–60.

Spigel DR, Hainsworth JD, Shipley DL, Ervin TJ, Kohler PC, Lubiner ET, et al. A randomized phase II trial of pemetrexed/gemcitabine/bevacizumab or pemetrexed/carboplatin/bevacizumab in the first-line treatment of elderly patients with advanced non-small cell lung cancer. *J. Thorac. Oncol.* 2012 janv;7(1):196–202.

Spiro SG, Rudd RM, Souhami RL, Brown J, Fairlamb DJ, Gower NH, et al. Chemotherapy versus supportive care in advanced non-small cell lung cancer: improved survival without detriment to quality of life. *Thorax.* 2004 oct;59(10):828–36.

Spratlin J. Ramucirumab (IMC-1121B): Monoclonal antibody inhibition of vascular endothelial growth factor receptor-2. *Curr. Oncol. Rep.* 2011 avr;13(2):97–102.

Steiner P, Joynes C, Bassi R, Wang S, Tonra JR, Hadari YR, et al. Tumor growth inhibition with cetuximab and chemotherapy in non-small cell lung cancer xenografts expressing wild-type and mutated epidermal growth factor receptor. *Clin. Cancer Res.* 2007 mars 1;13(5):1540–51.

Stockwin LH, Holmes S. Antibodies as therapeutic agents: vive la renaissance! *Expert Opin. Biol. Ther.* 2003 oct;3(7):1133–52.

Sullivan LA, Brekken RA. The VEGF family in cancer and antibody-based strategies for their inhibition. *MAbs.* 2010;2(2):165–75.

Takahashi H, Shibuya M. The vascular endothelial growth factor (VEGF)/VEGF receptor system and its role under physiological and pathological conditions. *Clin. Sci.* 2005 sept;109(3):227–41.

Tan AR, Moore DF, Hidalgo M, Doroshow JH, Poplin EA, Goodin S, et al. Pharmacokinetics of cetuximab after administration of escalating single dosing and weekly fixed dosing in patients with solid tumors. *Clin. Cancer Res.* 2006 nov 1;12(21):6517–22.

Tan D, Deeb G, Wang J, Slocum HK, Winston J, Wiseman S, et al. HER-2/neu protein expression and gene alteration in stage I-IIIA non-small-cell lung cancer: a study of 140 cases using a combination of high throughput tissue microarray, immunohistochemistry, and fluorescent in situ hybridization. *Diagn. Mol. Pathol.* 2003 déc;12(4):201–11.

Tanaka S, Sakamori Y, Niimi M, Hazama M, Kim YH, Yanagihara K. Design paper: a phase II study of bevacizumab and erlotinib in patients with non-squamous non-small cell lung cancer that is refractory or relapsed after 1-2 previous treatment (BEST). *Trials.* 2011;12:120.

Tateishi M, Ishida T, Kohdono S, Hamatake M, Fukuyama Y, Sugimachi K. Prognostic influence of the co-expression of epidermal growth factor receptor and c-erbB-2 protein in human lung adenocarcinoma. *Surg. Oncol.* 1994 avr;3(2):109–13.

Tesar DB, Björkman PJ. An intracellular traffic jam: Fc receptor-mediated transport of immunoglobulin G. *Curr. Opin. Struct. Biol.* 2010 avr;20(2):226–33.

Tzahar E, Waterman H, Chen X, Levkowitz G, Karunagaran D, Lavi S, et al. A hierarchical network of interreceptor interactions determines signal transduction by Neu differentiation factor/neuregulin and epidermal growth factor. *Mol. Cell. Biol.* 1996 oct;16(10):5276–87.

Vanhoefer U, Tewes M, Rojo F, Dirsch O, Schleucher N, Rosen O, et al. Phase I study of the humanized antiepidermal growth factor receptor monoclonal antibody EMD72000 in patients with advanced solid tumors that express the epidermal growth factor receptor. *J. Clin. Oncol.* 2004 janv 1;22(1):175–84.

Veikkola T, Karkkainen M, Claesson-Welsh L, Alitalo K. Regulation of angiogenesis via vascular endothelial growth factor receptors. *Cancer Res.* 2000 janv 15;60(2):203–12.

Vejle Hospital. First-line chemotherapy and panitumumab in advanced non-small cell lung cancer (Lung-TRIO). In: ClinicalTrials.gov [Internet]. Bethesda (MD): National Library of Medicine (US). 2000- [cited 2012 Feb 28]. Available from: http://clinicaltrials.gov /show/NCT01038037 NLM Identifier NCT01038037

Von Pawel J, Harvey JH, Spigel DR, Dediu M, Reck M, Cebotaru CL, Kumm E, Gallant G, Fox N and Camidge DR. A randomized phase II trial of mapatumumab, a TRAIL-R1 agonist monoclonal antibody, in combination with carboplatin and paclitaxel in patients with advanced NSCLC. *J. Clin. Oncol.* 2010;28(18s), (suppl; abstr LBA7501).

Vugmeyster Y, DeFranco D, Pittman DD, Xu X. Pharmacokinetics and lung distribution of a humanized anti-RAGE antibody in wild-type and RAGE-/- mice. *MAbs.* 2010 oct;2(5):571–5.

Wagenblast J, Hambek M, Baghi M, Gstöttner W, Strebhardt K, Ackermann H, et al. Antiproliferative activity of bortezomib alone and in combination with cisplatin or docetaxel in head and neck squamous cell carcinoma cell lines. *J. Cancer Res. Clin. Oncol.* 2008 mars;134(3):323–30.

Wakelee HA, Patnaik A, Sikic BI, Mita M, Fox NL, Miceli R, et al. Phase I and pharmacokinetic study of lexatumumab (HGS-ETR2) given every 2 weeks in patients with advanced solid tumors. *Ann. Oncol.* 2010 févr;21(2):376–81.

Waltenberger J, Claesson-Welsh L, Siegbahn A, Shibuya M, Heldin CH. Different signal transduction properties of KDR and Flt1, two receptors for vascular endothelial growth factor. *J. Biol. Chem.* 1994 oct 28;269(43):26988–95.

Ward ES, Ober RJ. Chapter 4: Multitasking by exploitation of intracellular transport functions the many faces of FcRn. *Adv. Immunol.* 2009;103:77–115.

Weiner LM, Belldegrun AS, Crawford J, Tolcher AW, Lockbaum P, Arends RH, et al. Dose and schedule study of panitumumab monotherapy in patients with advanced solid malignancies. *Clin. Cancer Res.* 2008 janv 15;14(2):502–8.

Wiley SR, Schooley K, Smolak PJ, Din WS, Huang CP, Nicholl JK, et al. Identification and characterization of a new member of the TNF family that induces apoptosis. *Immunity.* 1995 déc;3(6):673–82.

William WN Jr, Kies MS, Fossella FV, Liu DD, Gladish G, Tse WH, et al. Phase 2 study of carboplatin, docetaxel, and bevacizumab as frontline treatment for advanced nonsmall-cell lung cancer. *Cancer.* 2010 mai 15;116(10):2401–8.

Winter G, Harris WJ. Humanized antibodies. *Trends Pharmacol. Sci.* 1993 mai;14(5):139–43.

Xu N, Cai G, Ye W, Wang X, Li Y, Zhao P, et al. Molecular imaging application of radioiodinated anti-EGFR human Fab to EGFR-overexpressing tumor xenografts. *Anticancer Res.* 2009 oct;29(10):4005–11.

Yu L, Ju DW, Chen W, Li T, Xu Z, Jiang C, et al. 131I-chTNT radioimmunotherapy of 43 patients with advanced lung cancer. *Cancer Biother. Radiopharm.* 2006 févr;21(1):5–14.

Zhan P, Wang J, Lv X, Wang Q, Qiu L, Lin X, et al. Prognostic value of vascular endothelial growth factor expression in patients with lung cancer: a systematic review with meta-analysis. *J. Thorac. Oncol.* 2009 sept;4(9):1094–103.

Zhang D, Samani AA, Brodt P. The role of the IGF-I receptor in the regulation of matrix metalloproteinases, tumor invasion and metastasis. *Horm. Metab. Res.* 2003 déc;35(11-12):802–8.

Zhang L, Zhang X, Barrisford GW, Olumi AF. Lexatumumab (TRAIL-receptor 2 mAb) induces expression of DR5 and promotes apoptosis in primary and metastatic renal cell carcinoma in a mouse orthotopic model. *Cancer Lett.* 2007 juin 18;251(1):146–57.

Zinner RG, Glisson BS, Fossella FV, Pisters KMW, Kies MS, Lee PM, et al. Trastuzumab in combination with cisplatin and gemcitabine in patients with Her2-overexpressing, untreated, advanced non-small cell lung cancer: report of a phase II trial and findings regarding optimal identification of patients with Her2-overexpressing disease. *Lung Cancer.* 2004 avr;44(1):99–110.

Zinner RG, Saxman SB, Peng G, Monberg MJ, Ortuzar WI. Treatment rationale and study design for a randomized trial of pemetrexed/carboplatin followed by maintenance pemetrexed versus paclitaxel/carboplatin/bevacizumab followed by maintenance bevacizumab in patients with advanced non-small-cell lung cancer of nonsquamous histology. *Clin. Lung Cancer.* 2010 sept 1;11(5):352–7.

In: Non-Small Cell Lung Cancer: New Research
Editor: Lina Pasquariello

ISBN: 978-1-62417-804-7

Chapter 2

Non-coding RNAs (ncRNAs) in Non-Small Cell Lung Cancer (NSCLC)

Emanuela Bostjančič and Damjan Glavač*
Department of Molecular Genetics, Faculty of Medicine,
University of Ljubljana, Ljubljana, Slovenia

Abstract

Lung cancer is one of the most common cancers and non-small cell lung cancer (NSCLC) accounts for 80-85% of lung cancers. There are three main histological subtypes of NSCLC, adenocarcinoma (AD), squamous cell carcinoma (SCC) and large cell carcinoma (LCC), with a difference in survival rate between stage I and II. In addition, AD and SCC respond differently to certain treatments. The prognosis of NSCLC remains poor across all stages, despite advances in staging techniques and treatments. Emerging genomic technologies, especially high-throughput microarray studies, have shown potential in refining current NSCLC diagnosis, classification, prognosis and treatment approaches. Of 90 % of transcribed eukaryotic genomes, only 1-2 % encode for proteins, with the vast majority being non-coding RNAs (ncRNAs). ncRNAs are functional transcripts that do not code for proteins. They are predominantly composed of small double-stranded RNAs (dsRNAs) and are important regulators of gene expression in many eukaryotes. Three types of naturally occurring small RNAs have been described based on their origin or function: short interfering RNAs (siRNAs), repeat-associated short interfering RNAs (rasiRNAs) and microRNAs (miRNAs). Genome-wide profiling has shown that ncRNAs have distinct signatures specific for a certain cancer type. miRNAs are the most widely studied and characterized of all the ncRNAs. It is estimated that there could be as many as a thousand miRNAs, thought to regulate 30-90 % of genes within the human genome. Expression profiling of many microRNAs (miRNAs) in various normal and disease tissues has demonstrated unique spatial and temporal expression patterns. Moreover, global mean expression profiling in several studies has demonstrated differential expression of panels of miRNAs between AD and SCC, suggesting that they may be useful biomarkers for accurate classification of NSCLC. We will outline current knowledge about some specific ncRNAs and their

* Fax: + 386 1 543 7181. Phone: + 386 1 5437180. E-mail: damjan.glavac@mf.uni-lj.si.

predicted target genes in NSCLC and evaluate their potential as circulating biomarkers and therapeutic targets in NSCLC.

Serum miRNAs distinguish tumours from normal lung tissues and define the histology, growth rate and clinical outcome. Sputum can be used with highly sensitive and specific non-invasive markers for early detection of lung AD. miRNAs could play an important role in the design of innovative therapies for NSCLC. Studies have documented the implications of miRNAs in nearly all carcinogenesis processes. It has also been shown that miRNAs can be delivered systematically and can reduce invasion, proliferation and growth, as well as induce radiosensitivity and resistance. Combining information on ncRNAs with that on other types of biomarkers can improve cancer risk assessment, detection and prognosis of NSCLC.

Keywords: Non-small cell lung cancer, ncRNAs, miRNA, snoRNA, lncRNA

1. Introduction

Lung cancer is one of the most common cancers, and 80 % of lung cancers are histopathologically classified as non-small cell lung cancer (NSCLC). There are three main histological subtypes of NSCLC, adenocarcinoma (AD), squamous cell carcinoma (SCC), and large cell carcinoma (LCC), with the difference in survival rate between stage I and II. NSCLC is commonly diagnosed in the advanced stage and has limiting therapeutic options. AD and SCC respond differently to certain treatments. In early stage is treatment of choice surgery, with a five year overall survival of 40 %, but a majority of patients are at advanced disease stage at the time of diagnosis, which limits first line therapy and an expected survival of less than 8 months. The prognosis of NSCLC remains poor across all stages, despite advances in staging techniques and treatments. Although undergoing curative resection, nearly a third of patients with stage I NSCLC die of recurrent disease [1, 2].

Recent studies suggest that advanced stages of cancer are susceptible to molecular perturbations, and this could be applicable through delivery of non-coding RNAs (ncRNAs). ncRNAs are group of endogenous RNAs that function as regulators of gene expression. They are involved in physiological as well as pathological state [3].

2. ncRNA

Classification. Of 90 % of transcribed eukaryotic genomes, only 1-2 % encode for proteins, the vast majority being non-coding RNAs (ncRNAs) that are more or less functional transcripts. These ncRNA sequences are fulfilling a wide range of unexpected functions in eukaryotic biology. The ncRNA sequences are included in introns of protein-coding and non-coding transcripts. Introns represent at least 30 % of human genome, and it is simply not known what proportions of transcribed introns are subsequently processed into smaller functional RNAs [4]. Based on their function, ncRNAs can be divided in two groups: infrastructural, including ribosomal (rRNA), transfer (tRNA), small nuclear (snRNA) and small nucleolar RNAs (snoRNA), and regulatory, including microRNAs (miRNA), piwi-interacting (piRNA), small-interfering (siRNA), long non-coding and large intergenic non-coding (lncRNA in lincRNA, respectively), promoter-associated small RNA, repeat-associated short interfering (rasiRNA) and enhancer RNAs (eRNA). The regulatory ncRNAs are important regulators of gene expression in many eukaryotes [3, 5]. Based on length, the regulatory ncRNAs can be divided in two groups; larger than 200 nucleotides (nt) are lncRNA and lincRNA, smaller than 200 nt are others [3]. Small RNAs guide diverse cellular pathways, from chromosome architecture to stem cell maintenance, transcription, chromatin structure, genome integrity, and most commonly mRNA stability. Distinct classes of these small RNAs are distinguished by their origins [6]. Recent findings suggest that snoRNA not only have infrastructural function but have regulatory as well [3]. Some ncRNAs trigger different types of gene silencing that are collectively referred to as RNA silencing or RNA interference [7].

RNA interference (RNAi). RNAi is believed to be an evolutionary conserved mechanism in response to presence of dsRNA in the cell. A key step in the known silencing pathways is the processing of dsRNAs into short RNA duplexes of characteristic size and structure. The enzyme Dicer, which initiates the RNAi pathway, cleaves dsRNA to short double-stranded fragments of 20–25 base pairs (bp), named siRNA. siRNA possess perfect complementarity to the target gene mRNA, causing its degradation. RNAi is RNA-guided regulation of gene expression, historically known by other names, including post-transcriptional gene silencing. When the dsRNA is exogenous, coming from infection by a virus with RNA genome or laboratory manipulations, the RNA is imported directly into the cytoplasm where it is cleaved by the Dicer. The initiating dsRNA can also be endogenous, expressed from RNA-coding genes in the genome. Some of small RNAs are processed in a similar way or with components of RNAi pathway [6, 8-9].

Functional role. miRNAs are the most widely studied and characterized of all the ncRNAs. The roles of non-coding RNAs, other than miRNAs, in the regulation of transcription, such as epigenetic control of genes and repetitive sequences, are not as well understood. The contexts of gene regulation by ncRNAs in non-human systems were discussed and provided insights into how these processes could function in human cells. Regulatory ncRNAs are involved in development, response to stress and environmental stimuli, regulating chromatin remodelling, transcription (positive or negative impact), and post-transcription processing (splicing, transport, translation, degradation) [3].

Since the majority of research regarding NSCLC and ncRNAs was performed on miRNAs and in lesser extend on lncRNAs/lincRNAs and snoRNAs, will this review further focused on these three groups of ncRNAs.

2.1. miRNA

Genomic organization. miRNAs are genome encoded small (~ 20-22 nt), single-stranded ncRNAs, derived either from intergenic regions either from exon sequences of non-coding transcription units; but up to 60 % of known miRNAs are from intronic sequences of either protein coding or non-coding transcription units. They are encoded as a single gene or gene clusters. Some of miRNA clusters are co-regulated and co-transcribed. It has been predicted that miRNAs constitute more than 3 % of human genes [10]. Intergenic miRNAs are transcribed as an independent transcription unit, as a monocistronic, bicistronic or polycistronic primary transcript [11]. Intronic miRNA are preferentially transcribed in the same orientation as the host gene, probably not transcribed from their own promoters. They are processed from introns, as are many snoRNA. Intronic miRNAs and their host transcripts are co-regulated and co-transcribed from the same promoter [12]. Within the genome, there might be more than one copy of particular miRNAs. The suggestion has been made that some miRNAs are also encoded in antisense DNA, which is not transcribed to the mRNA [11].

MicroRNA biogenesis. Regulation of miRNA expression depends on transcription factors and epigenetic mechanisms. During maturation miRNAs undergo extensive post-transcriptional modifications. Genes encoding miRNAs are transcribed with RNA-polymerase II or RNA-polymerase III (Pol II or Pol III) into a long primary transcript (200 nt to several kilobases, kb), named *pri-miRNA*. The resulting *pri-miRNA* (containing poly-A tail and 7-methylguanosine cap) is processed in the nucleus by Drosha (RNase III enzyme). The resulting 70-nt stem-loop structure called *pre-miRNA* is imported into the cytoplasm by a transporter protein, Exportin 5. After GTP hydrolysis, with consequent release of the *pre-miRNA*, the double-stranded RNA portion of *pre-miRNA* is bound and cleaved by Dicer (RNase III enzyme). The action of these proteins removes the terminal loop and produces a miRNA:miRNA* duplex, which is a transient intermediate in miRNA biogenesis (20–25 nt). One of the two strands of each fragment is together with proteins argonaute (Ago 1-4), helicases, nucleases and RNA binding proteins, incorporated into a complex called the miRNA-containing ribonucleoprotein complex (miRNP). The resulting complex base-pair with complementary mRNA sequences. The other strand, miRNA*, is presumably degraded, although there are increasing evidence that either or both strands may be functional [10, 11, 13, 14]. Intronic miRNAs bypass Drosha cleavage and rely on the action of the *pre-mRNA* splicing/debranching machinery to produce an approx. 60 nt precursor miRNA hairpin (*pre-miRNA*) [12]. Numerous alternative pathways differing from canonical miRNA biogenesis pathways have been described recently and subset of several diverse longer non-coding RNAs can serve as precursors for miRNAs [15, 16]. Biogenesis of miRNA is represented in Figure 1.

MicroRNAs mechanism. The functional role of miRNA varies, but the primary mechanism of miRNA action in mammals is believed to be inhibition of mRNA translation by base-pairing to 3' UTR of target mRNA. The catalytic components of miRNP complex are Ago proteins. After base pairing between the miRNA and target mRNA either degradation of the target mRNA (perfect complementarity of miRNA:mRNA binding) either suppression of its translation occurs (when base pairing between these two molecules is incomplete).
Especially in animals, each miRNA can inhibit the translation of many different mRNAs, there could be as many as 200 predicted target genes per miRNA. In addition, mRNA can be regulated by more than one miRNA. The cooperative action of multiple identical (multiplicity) or different miRNPs (cooperativity) appears to provide the most efficient translational inhibition and additional mechanism to increase the specificity of miRNAs. Binding of single miRNA alone is usually insufficient to measurably block translation; combinatorial control of gene expression may be also provided by a set of co-ordinately expressed miRNAs [6]. Proteins or mRNA secondary structures could restrict miRNP accessibility to the UTRs, or may facilitate recognition of the authentic mRNA targets [10, 11, 13, 14].

Outcomes of miRNAs function. To the best of current knowledge, miRNAs mainly function as translational repressors and in normal cell conditions this may occur in different ways: (i) for mRNAs that should not be expressed in a particular cell type, the protein production is reduced to inconsequential levels (switch off the targets); (ii) miRNAs can adjust protein output for customized expression in different cell types (fine-tuning target expression); (iii) some miRNAs act as bystanders, where down-regulation by miRNAs is tolerated or reversed by feedback processes (neutral target expression) [11]. Role of miRNA can be further divided in three paradigms: combinatorial control (defined as cooperativity), cell-to-cell variation, and specific versus housekeeping functions [17]. There is still the prospect that some miRNA might specify more than just post-transcriptional repression; some might in addition target DNA for transcriptional silencing [11]. miRNAs may also target 5' UTR, open reading frames and even DNA sequences to regulate transcription, although translation repression was suggested as the predominant mechanism. miRNAs have been paradoxically also shown to up-regulate gene expression by enhancing translation under specific conditions [18].

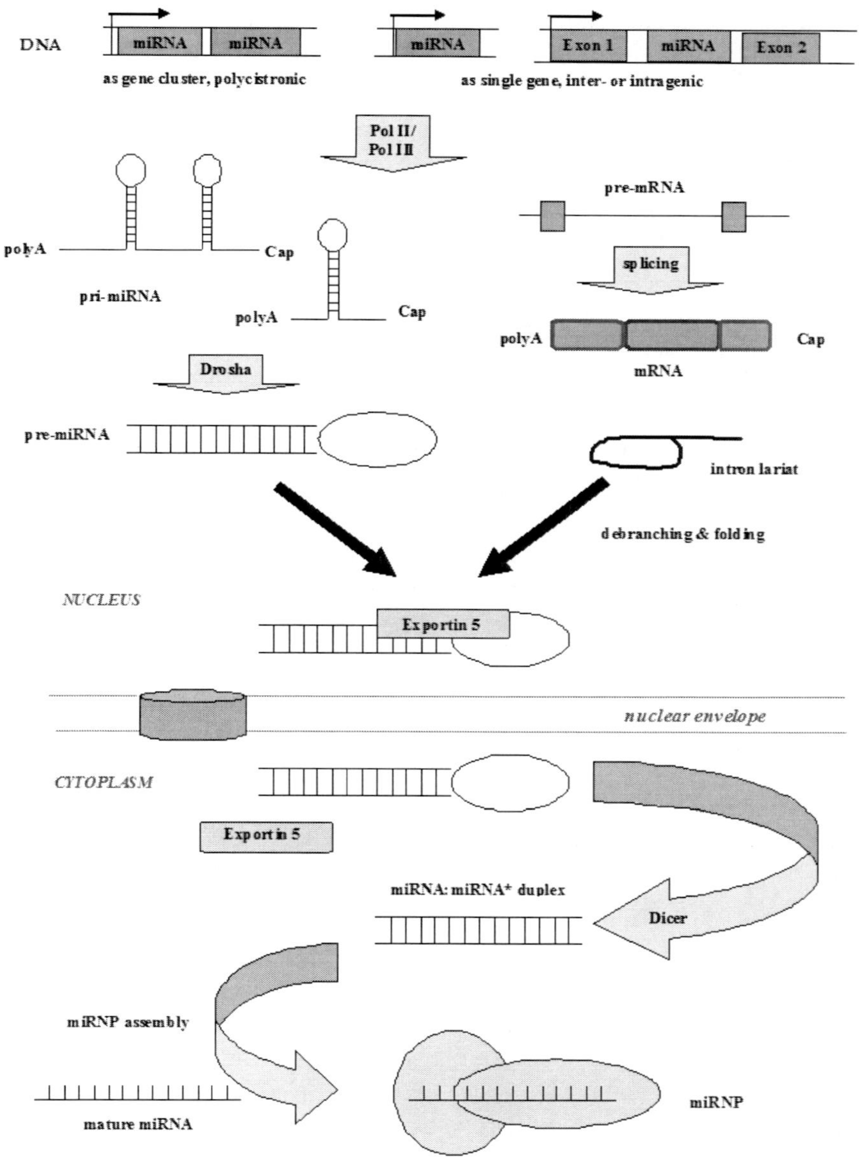

Figure 1. Schematic diagram of miRNA processing within the cell.

Biological function. Despite the large number of identified miRNAs, the scope of their roles in regulating cellular gene expression is not fully understood. Most known functions of miRNAs relate to negative gene regulation, thought to regulate 30-90 % of genes within the human genome. Expression profiling of many microRNAs (miRNAs) in various normal and disease tissues has demonstrated unique spatial and temporal expression patterns. Many miRNAs are expressed in a tissue-specific manner and/or cell-type specific manner; they are important at distinct stages of development and have been found to regulate a variety of developmental and physiological processes [8]. miRNAs are involved in a myriad of biological processes, including proliferation, apoptosis, metabolism, differentiation and epithelial-mesenchymal-transition (EMT), regulation of insulin secretion, stem cell division and development, proper organ formation, embryonic pattering and body growth, cholesterol metabolism, resistance to viral infection and oxidative stress, immune response etc [2, 8]. With all different genes and expression patterns, it is reasonable to propose that every cell type at each developmental stage might have a distinct miRNA expression profile.

Defining miRNA targets and databases. In addition to identifying reciprocally regulated miRNA-mRNA, many computational methods have been recently developed for identifying potential miRNA targets [19]. Most of these methods search for multiple conserved regions of miRNA complementarities within 3' UTR; the most important parameters are therefore evolutionary conservation with regard to the quality and stability of base pairing and predicted binding energy. The interaction between seven consecutive nucleotides in the target mRNAs 3' UTR and the 1-8 nt ("seed sequence") at the 5' miRNA end is believed to be important for base pairing. The majority of prediction programmes use pairing with the seed sequence as one of the major criteria. There are several available programs for predicting mRNA targets for specific miRNA, but none of these programs can be used as a means of independently validating the targets, and all predicted targets must be validated *in vitro* and *in vivo* [20]. Further complicating target site prediction in mammals is the fact that not all 3' UTR sites with perfect complementarities to the miRNA seed nucleotides are functional. Moreover, mRNAs sites with imperfect seed complementarities can themselves be very good miRNA targets. Bioinformatic analysis is therefore much noisier and more prone to false positive and false negative predictions [21]. There is also a database available containing deregulated miRNAs in different diseases or their profiling in various tissues (HMDD, Human MicroRNA Disease Database) [22]. To date, almost 2000 human miRNAs have been identified, all are collected in miRBase [23].

2.2. SnoRNA

Classification. Small ncleolar RNAs (snoRNAs) are group of single-stranded RNAs generally of ~ 60-300 nt in length. Based on conserved nucleotide motifs, snoRNAs are classified into two distinct families: box C/D (60–200 nt) and box H/ACA (120-250 nt). Each snoRNA family recruits specific set of effectors proteins to form functional snoRNA ribonucleoproteins (snoRNPs). Two main classes differ in terms of sequence and structural elements, binding partners and nature of chemical modification catalysed; box C/D snoRNA drives 2'-O-ribose methylation, and box H/ACA drives pseudouridylation. Subset of snoRNA termed small Cajal RNAs (scaRNAs) are specifically localizes to Cajal bodies. Cajal bodies are place of post-transcriptional modification (covalent modification) of small nuclear RNAs (snRNAs), snoRNAs and assembly of snoRNA in mature snoRNP [15]. ScaRNA conform the C/D-H/ACA classification, some containing structural motifs characteristic of both snoRNA families [15, 24].

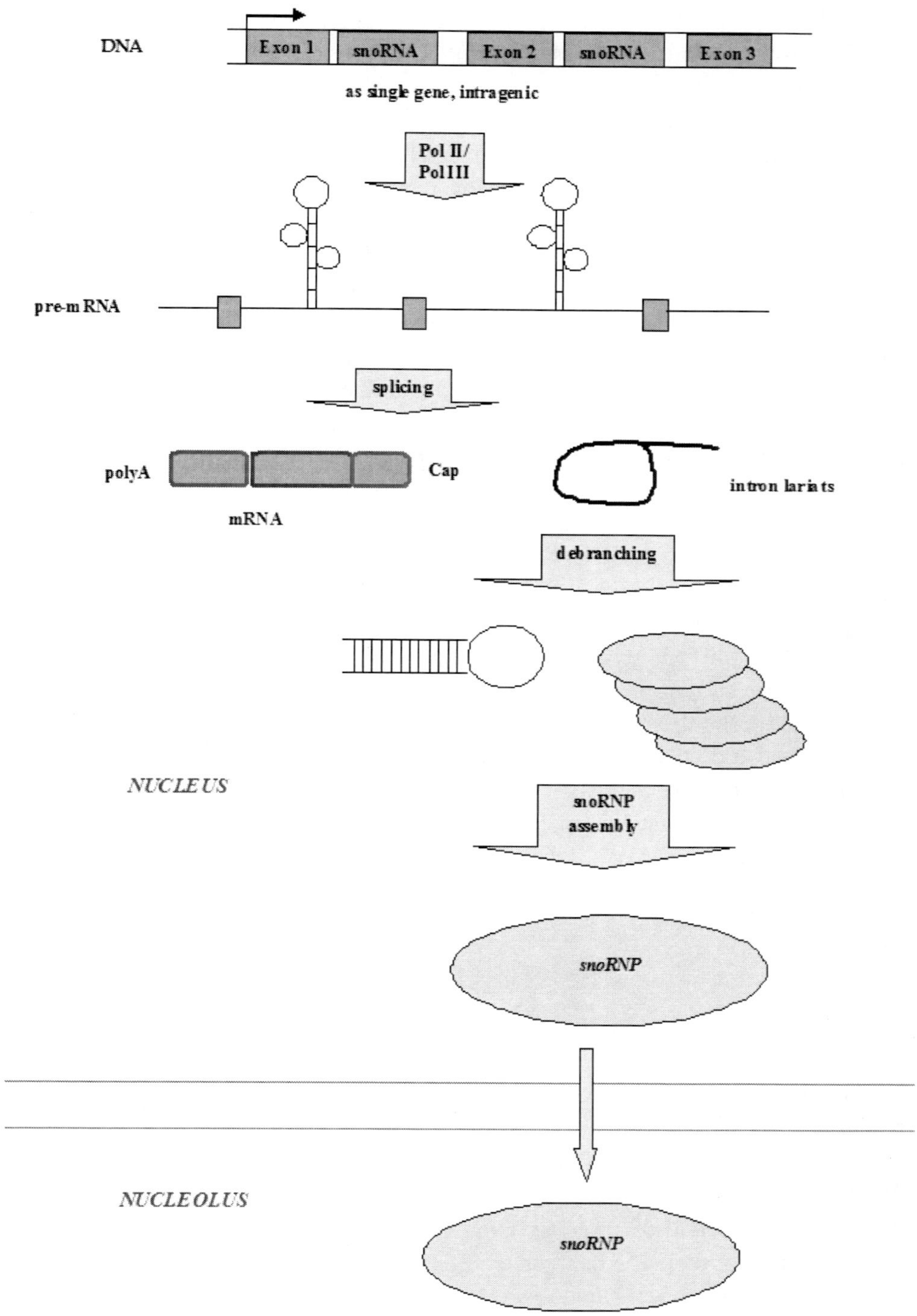

Figure 2. Schematic diagram of snoRNA processing within the cell.

Biogenesis. snoRNAs encoding genes display diverse organization patterns in different organisms; they mostly arise from introns excised from protein or non-protein coding transcripts (and are co-transcribed with the host gene transcript), but can be also transcribed from independent promoters with Pol II or Pol III (as individually genes or form polycistronic clusters) [15]. Following transcription, snoRNA-containing introns are removed from pre-mRNA by the spliceosome, which contains snRNAs, the targets of scaRNA. snoRNAs are processed from introns by RNAase III like activity. Maturation process includes snoRNA transition through Cajal bodies, where they are chemically modified and further transported to the nucleolus, where they are typically localized. The biogenesis of snoRNAs is summarized in Figure 2, but is less well understood then biogenesis of miRNAs [18, 24].

snoRNA function. Located in the nucleolus, they are best known as guide molecules for 2'-O-ribose methylation or pseudouridylation (isomerisation of uridine) of specific RNA nucleotides.A few are required for pre-rRNA endonucleolytic processing – rRNA and snRNA modification. Several snoRNAs are expressed in tissue specific region. It was recently shown, that in addition to its canonical function, they also participate in regulation of alternative splicing and antisense type mechanism, therefore influencing gene expression. SnoRNA-guided modifications of mRNAs could affect splicing, translation, or mRNA stability, but this area is more or less unstudied.In addition to these roles related to classical snoRNAs functions, numerous orphan snoRNAs have been transcribed, with no known target [18, 24]. A growing body of evidence suggests that many snoRNAs can also give rise to other regulatory RNA species, like miRNA. These sno-derived RNAs (sdRNA) are produced from double-stranded snoRNA structures by the components of RNAi pathway; sdRNAs also interact with Argonaute proteins, displaying miRNA capabilities [15, 24].

Database. All published human snoRNA sequences and annotating data are stored in the snoRNABase. The current version 3 contains 402 experimentally confirmed human snoRNAs. It is proposed that total number of sno-RNA like sequences in the human genome may be greater than 1000 [24].

miRNAs and snoRNAs share similarities in processing pathways and protein interaction partners, sub-cellular localization (a large proportion of human mature miRNAs have been detected in the nucleus as well as a subset of small RNAs derived from snoRNAs have been detected in the cytoplasm), genomic organization and location, as well as levels of conservation [15].

2.3. Long Non-Coding RNA

Classification and genomic organization. Long non-coding RNA (lncRNAs) are those greater than 200 nt, apparently the most numerous and functionally diverse. It is estimated that number of new unexplored lncRNA transcripts is ~ 15000. Approx. one third to one half of lncRNAs overlap protein-coding loci in some way, giving importance for lncRNA annotation since thousands of protein-coding genes harbour natural antisense transcripts belonging to the lncRNAs. Large intergenic ncRNAs (lincRNAs), a class of ncRNAs, tend to be modestly conserved; they both up- and down- regulate hundreds of gene expression. Further, 25 % of enhancers co-localize with RNAPII site, suggesting that some enhancers RNAs are also transcribed; these transcripts are termed eRNAs for enhancer RNAs. It have not been yet defined whether the activating lncRNAs are in fact a subset of such eRNAs [25].

Function. They are key regulators of epigenetic gene regulation in mammalian cells [25]. Many of the identified lncRNAs show spatial- and temporal-specific patterns of expression. Generally lncRNAs have been implicated in gene-regulatory roles, such as chromatin dosage-compensation, imprinting, epigenetic regulation, cell cycle control, nuclear and cytoplasmic trafficking, transcription, translation, splicing, cell differentiation etc. Almost every step in the life cycle of genes (transcription, mRNAs splicing, RNA decay, translation) can be influenced by lncRNAs [26].

Database. The lncRNA database provides sequence, structural, and conservation evidence for multi-species lncRNAs, together with a list of lncRNAs that are experimentally known to interact with coding mRNAs [25].

3. ncRNA and Cancer

Biological role of ncRNAs in cancer. ncRNAs have been recognized as gene-specific regulators and are similar in activity to a large number of protein transcription factors that are known to be critical in the transformation of cells to a malignant state. These RNAs can regulate every stage of gene expression: transcription, mRNA stability, and mRNA translation. Cancer cells have genetic and epigenetic changes from their normal counterparts and the role of ncRNAs in mediating these differences is beginning to emerge. Genome-wide profiling has shown that ncRNAs have distinct signatures specific for a certain cancer type. Importance of combining ncRNAs with other biomarkers for cancer detection and prognosis would improve cancer risk assessment, detection, and prognosis. Specific genetic polymorphisms are associated with the risk of developing several types of cancer. Thus, there is a need to combine genomic mutations with ncRNA markers to develop marker panels for more accurate risk assessment and early diagnosis [3, 5, 26].

Significance of early detection of preneoplastic lesions. Genome-wide profiling have examined miRNAs in preneoplasias or their usefulness to predict progression from preneoplasia to cancer. Several lines of evidence suggest (i) the potential usefulness of ncRNAs, particularly miRNAs, as signatures of early events in carcinogenesis and as biomarkers in early cancer detection; (ii) as differential indicators of benign lesions, preneoplasia, and neoplasia; (iii) that miRNAs and perhaps other ncRNAs might be useful in determining which preneoplastic lesions are likely to progress to cancer. Distinguishing benign diseases and certain non-precancerous lesions from precancerous lesions and metastatic tumours, would improve patient outcomes and survival, reduce patient discomfort, and reduce costs [27].

3.1. miRNAs

miRNAs are thought to regulate a quarter of all mammalian genes and alterations in their expression have been associated with the development of cancer. Establishing the nature of gene regulation by microRNAs during normal development and physiology will be vital to understanding their role in cancer [28]. miRNAs have been shown to be up- or down-regulated in a wide variety of human cancers, suggesting a role for miRNAs in tumorigenesis.

miRNAs can act as both tumour-suppressor genes and oncogenes. There are different ways in which miRNAs appear to be involved in cancer: as tumour-suppressors, as oncogenes, or as agents involved in affecting genome stability. miRNAs appear to function as a tumour suppressor because a reduced function of the corresponding miRNA lead to elevated expression of potential oncogenes or processes, such as proliferation or reduced processes such as apoptosis. The increased expression of oncogenic miRNAs (oncomirs) appears to act in a manner analogous to an oncogene. Oncomirs are presumed to function by down-regulating tumour suppressor genes [17, 29].

Usefulness of miRNAs as potential biomarkers. MicroRNAs may serve as potential biomarkers for cancer diagnosis, prognosis and targets for therapy. As potential markers for diagnosis are better classification factors than mRNA [27, 28]. As potential markers for prognosis are miRNAs useful as markers for treatment response, for predicting progression, metastasis and survival. As biomarkers for therapy would be miRNAs useful as oncogenes, tumour-suppressors, stem cells, invasion and metastasis, and drug sensitivity [30]. Some of the key features of miRNAs that make them useful as potential biomarkers can be briefly summarized. (i) The expression patterns of miRNAs in human cancers appear to be tissue specific. (ii) miRNA profiles appear to reflect developmental lineage and differentiation state of the tumours. (iii) miRNAs can successfully classify poorly differentiated tumours with high accuracy (~ 70%).

In contrast, mRNA profiles in the same set of specimens had an accuracy of only 6 %. Therefore, a combination of both miRNA and mRNA profiling data has the potential of enhancing accuracy of tumour classification. (iv) miRNAs are stable in human body fluids of plasma and serum. (v) miRNAs can be quantitatively measured in microliter quantities of human sera or plasma using qPCR. (vi) miRNAs can also be profiled and quantitatively measured in formalin-fixed tissues [27, 28, 31].

Mutations and epigenetics. Mutations that have been identified to cause cancer in humans and in mouse models of human cancer have solidified the roles of miRNA in malignancy. Disruption of miRNA target interaction in the form of single-nucleotide polymorphisms (SNPs), either in the miRNA gene or its target site (3′ UTR mRNA), can lead to complete gain or loss of the miRNA function and thus account for a diseased state. In contrast to the miRNA target sites in mRNA transcripts, in which the potential of variation is huge, variants identified in miRNA sequences tend to be extremely rare, usually restricted to one individual. The presence of SNPs in *pri-miRNA* or *pre-miRNA* can also affect the processing of miRNAs, their expression and/or binding to target mRNA [21].

Approx. half of miRNA genes are encoded in genomic region prone to cancer-associated genomic regions or in fragile chromosomal sites that are often associated with rearrangements in cancer cells [1, 17]. Recent advances in miRNA research have provided evidence of a miRNA association with epigenetic mechanisms activated in diseased human tissues. Also lncRNA have already been implicated in human diseases such as cancer and neurodegeneration [25].

Multiple studies have identified small- and large-scale mutations affecting noncoding regions of the genome, including chromosomal translocation, copy-number variation, nucleotide expansion, and SNPs, linking distinct types of mutations in lncRNA genes with diverse diseases [26].

4. ncRNA and NSCLC

IGDB.NSCLC is an integrated genomic database of NSCLC. It includes data to illustrate genomic alteration (chromosomal regions with copy number alteration, gain- and loss-of-function studies, LOH), aberrant expressed genes and miRNAs, somatic mutation, experimental evidence and clinical information of alterations [32]. In Table 1 are summarized some miRNAs with known targets in NSCLC.

4.1. miRNA and NSCLC

4.1.1. Current Understanding of Aberrantly Expressed miRNAs in NSCLC, Their Target Genes, and Usefulness as Prognostic Factors

Based on cell line and animal models as well as human tissue and xenografts, the miRNAs have a potential as prognostic, therapeutic and diagnostic biomarkers in NSCLC. There is increasing evidence that altered miRNAs expression, mutational status, presence/absence of SNP and methylation, are associated with NSCLC progression and survival, invasive, aggressive and metastatic tumour capabilities, resistance and higher risk of relapse, tumour differentiation, pathological stage and lymph-node metastasis, and are as well important as early stage prognostic biomarker, oncogenes, tumour-suppressor, therapeutic and diagnostic targets. miRNAs significantly distinguish: tumours from normal lung tissues, tumour histology and growth rate, clinical outcome and year of lung cancer detection. Results indicate a role for miRNAs in lung tissues and plasma as molecular predictors of lung cancer development and aggressiveness and have strong clinical implication both for lung cancer management and in the clinical laboratory [2].

Dicer. The significance of miRNAs in NSCLC is displayed by decreased Dicer expression [8]; lower Dicer expression was an independent prognostic indicator for surgically treated NSCLC [1], its reduced expression was associated with poor prognosis [33]. In contrast, Dicer was shown to be up-regulated in precursor lesions of lung AD, higher Dicer expression was also detected in SCC compared to AD. Fractions of AD lose Dicer due to deletions of the Dicer locus [34].

Hypoxia. Hypoxia is an essential feature of neoplastic microenvironment; tumours with extensive low oxygen tend to exhibit poor prognosis and resistance to conventional therapy. Hypoxia-inducible factors (HIFs) are well documented master regulators of response to low oxygen. HIF orchestrates the expression of variety of genes, critical for adaptation to low oxygen. In hypoxia, the HIF stabilization leads to activation of a hundred of genes that regulate angiogenesis, glucose metabolism, migration, survival and death, slow down or arrest of the cell cycle. HIF can also function as transcriptional repressor. A group of hypoxia regulated miRNAs has been identified, providing an additional link between a tumour specific factor and gene expression control. Most hypoxia induced miRNAs are over-expressed in human cancers. In case of hypoxia regulated miRNAs, a highly complex spectrum of candidate targets is defined, including genes involved in proliferation, apoptosis, DNA repair, chromatin remodelling, metabolism and migration [35]. Additional transcription factors that under certain conditions respond to hypoxia/anoxia, such as p53 in NF-Kb, have been shown to affect the expression of selected miRNAs [36]. One of miRNA regulated by hypoxia, miR-210, was shown to be over-expressed at late stages of NSCLC, to cause an alteration of cell viability in AD cell lines, and to induce a loss of mitochondrial membrane potential, therefore suggesting its impact on cell metabolism, survival and modulation of HIF-1 activity [37].

Apoptosis and p53. Several independent studies have shown that miR-34 is an important component of the p53 tumour suppressor network; p53 is a target for members of miR-34 family, while miR-34 is often up-regulated in cells expressing p53 or following p53 activation and DNA damage. Up-regulation of miR-34a by p53 results in an enhanced reduction in cell proliferation, therefore suggesting reinforcement of tumour suppressor function of p53 by miR-34a and promotion of apoptosis [8]. Three members of miR-34 family are known to have role in human cancers, miR-34a, and miR-34b in miR-34c. MicroRNA, miR-34a is lost or down-regulated in many tumours, its over-expression leads to activation of apoptosis, indicating tumour suppressor role [2]. Expression of miR-34 family is down-regulated in NSCLC compared to normal tissue and related to higher-risk of relapse [38]. miR-34b, miR-34c and miR-449 are enriched in only few tissues including lung and trachea; reduced expression of miR-34c together with another 4 miRNAs correlated with poor survival of SCC patients [2]. In another panel of NSCLC tissues, miR-34a and miR-199a/b were found to be down-regulated and significantly co-expressed. A lower expression of all three miRNAs was associated with SCC, whereas NSCLC patients with miR-34 up-regulation showed a positive correlation with a longer survival [39].

Angiogenesis. In NSCLC patients, following the miRNA microarray analysis, gene enrichment analysis were performed, and the resulting enriched miRNAs were angiogenesis-related miRNAs. Significantly altered angiogenesis related miRNAs were: miR-21, miR-106a, miR-126, miR-155, miR-182, miR-210 and miR-424 [40]. As another angiogenesis-related miRNAs are defined, miR-221 and miR-222. High expression of miR-221 and miR-222 blocks angiogenesis and proliferation in endothelial cells, but they promote proliferation in cancer cells by targeting cell cycle inhibitor p27, suggesting that regulation of proliferation by these miRNAs is specific to cell type. Both, miR-221 and miR-222**,** are over-expressed in aggressive NSCLC and function by targeting PTEN and TIMP3, consequently enhance cellular migration. Oncogene c-MET was shown to be involved in miR-221 and miR-222 activation [2]. Further, miR-15b and miR-16 are down-regulated in hypoxic conditions of carcinoma cell line, which contributes to an increase in VEGF-mediated angiogenesis and induction of apoptosis [41]. Both were shown to be frequently down-regulated or deleted in NSCLC and are inversely correlated with Cyclin D1. It was shown that cell cycle arrest, induced by miR-15/miR-16 depends on expression of Rb, confirming that certain cyclins are major targets for these two miRNAs in NSCLC [42]. Recent findings demonstrated that miR-34a and miR-15a/16 are co-regulated in NSCLC and act synergistically to induce cell cycle arrest in Rb-dependent manner. No synergistic effect of these miRNAs was observed for apoptosis. As target, unique to miR-15a/16, Cyclin E1 was shown [43]. When patients with NSCLC were classified in three groups according to their miR-16 expression levels, those with normal levels had the best outcome, whereas those with high levels had the worst. These results indicate that miR-16 expression levels may serve as prognostic marker in NSCLC [44]. A tumour angiogenesis promoting activity has been attributed also to the miRNA cluster, miR-17-92, let-7f and miR-27b [2]. Using lung cancer cell lines, HIF-1 was shown to be a target for miR-17-92 [45]. MicroRNA cluster, miR-17-92 act as oncogene, it is involved in regulation of angiogenesis, it is induced by VEGF and its disruption may cause lethal abnormalities [2]. Further, the 3' UTR of VEGF possess a binding site for miR-126, an angiogenic miRNA. MicroRNA miR-126 was also shown to inhibit invasion in NSCLC cell lines [46]. Expression of miR-126 was down-regulated in eight lung cancer cell lines, and may alter lung cancer cell invasive capacity and growth [2]. High miR-126 expression correlated significantly with high VEGF-A expression in NSCLC. In addition, miR-126 was shown as significant negative prognostic factor [47].

Immunity. Numerous investigations have supported the role of miRNAs in the initiation and progression of human cancer, as well as in physiological function such as immune response, cell proliferation, cell death, and inflammation, which are also known to be regulated by NF-kB. NF-kB signalling cascades are critical to tumour development and malignant progression [48]. There is increasing evidence that miR-146a is involved in the regulation of the innate immune response. Numerous studies showed the induction of miR-146a expression by pro-inflammatory mediators. Expression of certain EBV protein induces miR-146a, and this aberrant miR-146a expression might be linked to cancerous phenotypes. miR-146a is either elevated either reduced in several types of cancers. The action of miR-146a is mediated through down-regulation of the NF-kB pathway. Activation of NF-kB in promoting the survival and metastatic potentials of cancer cells is widely accepted, since chronic inflammation and activation of NF-kB is associated with development of multiple cancers. It has been suggested that increase in miR-146a expression might be linked to cancer through inappropriate regulation of the inflammatory response, speculating that miR-146a mediated immune suppression might lead to increased survival of cancerous cells [49]. Indeed, miR-146a can suppress the metastatic ability of certain cancer types partially through decreasing constitutive NF-kB activity. miR-146a transduction inhibits invasion, migration and metastatic ability of metastasis cells [50]. In human lung alveolar epithelial tumour cells, IL-beta induces miR-146a and negatively regulates the release of IL-8 and RANTES, both of which are regulated by NF-kB activation, suggesting negative feedback regulation of inflammation following activation of the innate immune response. This is observed only at high IL-beta concentrations, indicating important feedback mechanism during severe inflammation [48]. In human NSCLC, miR-146b-3p and miR-146b-5p expressions were higher in stroma than in cancerous epithelia, and higher miR-146b-5p but lower miR-146b-3p expression was predictive of recurrence [51]. Another miRNA involved in regulation of immune response, is miR-155. Most recent publications on miR-155 support a positive correlation between miR-155 up-regulation and NF-kB activation. MicroRNA miR-155 is up-regulated in solid tumours of lung [48]. High expression of miR-155 and low expression of let-7a-2 were strongly associated with poor survival of patients with lung AD [2]. Furthermore, miR-155 was shown as prognostic marker and its impact depends on histological subtype and nodal status in NSCLC [52].

EMT (epithelial-to-mesenchymal-transition). The role of EMT miRNAs (miR-200b, miR-200c, miR-205) has been studied also in NSCLC carcinogenesis. These miRNAs were implicated in the dedifferentiation program in primary lung tumours after exposure to tobacco carcinogens [2]. In NSCLC cell lines, it was shown that expressions of miR-200c as well as E-kadherin are low in contrast to normal human bronchial epithelial cells. Since down-regulation of E-kadherin is a crucial event in EMT, loss of miR-200c could play a significant role in the initiation of an invasive phenotype, and equally, miR-200c over-expression holds potential for its reversal [53]. Lower miR-200c expression was also observed in NSCLC, and was associated with poor grade of differentiation and higher propensity to lymph node metastases. Therefore, loss of miR-200c expression induces aggressive, invasive and chemo-resistant phenotype [54]. Another miRNA involved in EMT is miR-30a. It inhibits EMT by targeting Snai1, a known modulator of EMT, and is down-regulated in NSCLC. Expression of miR-30a was found to be inversely proportional to invasive potential of various NSCLC cell lines. It was down-regulated in 81 % of patients with NSCLC compared to normal tissue [55].

Correlation between EGFR and miRNAs. Mutations in EGFR gene are more frequent in NSCLC patients who never smoked tobacco; a significant down-regulation of miR-145 has been demonstrated in the cancer tissues of these patients. Restoration of this miRNA can inhibit cancer cell growth in EGFR mutant lung AD [56]. Further, miR-146a transduction down-regulates expression of EGFR [50]. EGFR promotes lung tumorigenesis also by activating miR-7 expression. EGFR activation occurs commonly in lung cancer with poor prognosis. Characterization of an oncomir miR-7 and its role as a mediator of EGFR signalling in lung cancer cell was established, suggesting that miR-7 may act as important modulator of EGFR-mediated oncogenesis [57]. In NSCLC cell lines, miR-7 was reduced, its over-expression suppressed NSCLC cells proliferation, induced cell apoptosis, inhibited cell migration, and reduced tumorigenicity. As miR-7 target, Bcl-2 was demonstrated and was down-regulated by miR-7 at transcriptional and translational level [58].

miRNAs let-7. The let-7 family cluster is consisted of miRNAs genes mapped to different chromosomal regions that are frequently deleted in lung tumours. Reduced expression of let-7 in patients with lung AD has been correlated with poor prognosis [59]. In human lung cancers, let-7 expression decrease (> 50 %) correlate with the markedly elevated expression of RAS proteins; the cancer growth inhibitory activity was proposed for let-7 [1]. Let-7 acts as a tumour suppressor in lung cancers [30], negatively regulates RAS, MYC, HMGA2 and cyclins, its down-regulation is characteristic of NSCLC [1, 2]. Let-7g expression is absent in NSCLC cells and its aberrant expression is associated with the poor prognosis of lung cancer compared to normal lung cell. Potential role of pre-let-7g in lung cancer cell metastasis was evaluated and it is suggested that it could be suitable target for the suppression of lung cancer cell migration [60].

miRNA miR-21. There is an omnipresent over-expression of miR-21 in all types of human carcinomas, including lung cancers. NF-kB activation has been reported in all of these cancers, underscoring the interplay of miR-21 over-expression and NF-kB activation in cancer. Cell type specificity may cause the difference of miR-21 and NF-kB activity. As an example, in NSCLC miR-21 down-regulates PTEN and stimulates growth and invasion [61], in epithelial cell the same action results in increase of NF-kB activation. In LPS-stimulated macrophages miR-21 negatively regulates PDCD4 and activates NF-kB; however, during earlier stages of liver regeneration, miR-21 down-regulate activator of NF-kB, and works as NF-kB inhibitor [48]. Over-expression of mature miR-21 was shown as independent negative prognostic factor for overall survival in NSCLC. Increased miR-21 expression is associated with disease progression and survival in stage I lung cancer, giving it a potential as an early stage prognostic biomarker for lung AD. Changes in expression of miR-21 are more remarkable in the presence of EGFR mutations [62]. miR-21 enhances tumorigenesis, its genetic deletion partially protects against tumour formation and it drives tumorigenesis through inhibition of apoptosis [63].

Other analysed miRNAs with predicted prognostic value. MicroRNAs miR-451 was shown to be down-regulated in NSCLC tissue; its expression was significantly correlated with tumour differentiation, pathological stage and negatively correlated with lymph-node metastasis, and the stage of TNM classification. Its low expression is correlated to shorter survival of NSCLC patients and poor prognosis. As its target, RAB14 was proposed; over-expression inhibited cell cycle progression, cellular migration and invasive ability of NSCLC [64-65]. Combined analysis revealed that poor prognosis was associated with reduced let-7 and miR-122 level and increased miR-137, miR-372 and miR-182 level [1, 2]. Expression of miR-130a has been shown as increased in NSCLC and its over-expression was strongly associated with lymph node metastasis, stage of tumour node metastasis classification and poor prognosis. Difference was also shown between smoking and non-smoking patients. It was suggested as independent prognostic factor for patients with NSCLC [66]. MicroRNA miR-218 was found to be deleted and down regulated in lung SCC and was suggested as potential tumour suppressor [67]. PXN gene mutations are associated with lung AD, and PXN was shown as a target for miR-218. Expressions of PXN and miR-218 were tested for an overall survival and relapse-free survival, and might independently predict both. PXN was negatively regulated by miR-218 and cell proliferation and invasion were enhanced by PXN over-expression induced by miR-218 suppression [68]. Expression of miR-125a-3p and miR-125a-5p was lower in NSCLC tissue than in adjacent normal lung tissue. Correlation between their expression and pathological stage of lymph node metastasis was shown, as well as that they function in an opposing manner suppressing or enhancing cell migration and invasion [69]. MicroRNA miR-206 showed inverse correlation with metastatic potential of lung cancer, since it over-expression inhibited migration and invasion of lung cancer cells [70]. MicroRNA miR-328 was suggested as promising biomarker for differentiating patients with NSCLC who may and may not develop brain metastasis. Expression of miR-328 and miR-330-3p correctly classify these two groups of patients, while miR-328 has a role in conferring migratory potential to NSCLC [71]. Differential expression of miR-378 is associated with NSCLC brain metastasis by promoting cell migration invasion and tumour angiogenesis [72]. Low expression of miR-374a was shown as prognostic marker, since its down-regulation in early stage of NSCLC is associated with poor survival of patients [73]. In another research, clinical and pathological characteristics were examined, defining low expression level of miR-143 in correlation with smoking status and high miR-21 and low miR-181a level in correlation with poor survival among NSCLC patients. These three miRNAs were suggested as a novel diagnostic or prognostic biomarker for NSCLC [74].

Other analysed miRNAs. MicroRNA miR-133b was shown as regulator for MCL-1 and Bcl-2 in lung AD cell lines; its over-expression induces apoptosis [75]. MicroRNA miR-197 is expressed at higher levels in NSCLC; its elevated expression is correlated to reduced Fus-1 protein, which possesses tumour-suppressor function. Fus-1 is highly regulated at various levels, leading to lost or greatly diminished tumour suppressor function in many lung cancers [76]. MicroRNA miR-212 was found as negative regulator of PED, protein with an anti-apoptotic activity [77]. Its over-expression in NSCLC cells promoted cell cycle progression, cell proliferation, cell migration and invasion and that might have tumour-promoting properties being involved in tumorigenesis. Tumour suppressor PTCH1 was defined as functional target of miR-212 [78]. MicroRNA miR-101 inhibits cell proliferation and invasion in NSCLC, at least partially by repressing its targets EZH2 [79]. It was shown that miR-145 inhibits proliferation of NSCLC through c-Myc [80].

SNPs impact on miRNAs function. A single nucleotide polymorphism (SNP) in let-7 complementary site of KRAS mRNA 3' UTR has been found significantly associated with an increased risk of NSCLC [81]. Changes in expression of miR-146a miRNA could be related to a common polymorphism G/C (rs2910164) located in miR-146a [49]. The association between the presence of SNP in miR-196a2 and survival in individuals with NSCLC was shown as well as that this SNP affects binding of mature miRNA to its target mRNA [82]. Further, genetic variants in the pre-miRNA flanking region were found as potential prognostic biomarker of NSCLC [83].

Epigenetic impact on miRNA function. Aberrant miRNA gene methylation might contribute to the human cancer epigenome. MicroRNA family miR-29 (miR-29a/b/c) has been reported to be down-regulated in NSCLC and has complementarities to DNA methyltransferase (DNMT)-3A and -3B. The expression of miR-29s is inversely correlated to DNMT3A and -3B in lung cancer tissues and miR-29s directly targets both of the enzymes. Enforced expression of miR-29s restores normal pattern of DNA methylation, induces expression of methylation-silenced tumour suppressor genes and inhibits tumorigenesis, suggesting a role of miR-29s in the epigenetic normalization of NSCLC [84]. Let-7a-3 is found heavily methylated in normal lung cells, but hypomethylated and expressed in a subset of lung AD. Let-7a-3 hypomethylation facilitated epigenetic reactivation of the gene and its elevated expression, which results in enhanced tumour phenotypes and oncogenic transcription profiles. Let-7a-3 is therefore epigenetically regulated miRNA with oncogenic function [85].

Since miR-34a was down-regulated in NSCLC and low levels were correlated with higher probability of relapse, authors further investigated and found a relation between methylation of MIR34A promoter region and miR-34a expression [38]. Promoter hypermethylation of miR-34b/c was defined as relatively common event in NSCLC, and might be a potential prognostic factor for stage I NSCLC. Aberrant DNA methylation of miR-34b/c was correlated with a high probability of recurrence and associated with poor overall survival and disease-free survival [86]. For miR-9 and miR-193a, a tumour specific methylation was found in NSCLC patients. The shorter free survival of miR-9-3 methylated SCC patients compared to miR-9-3 unmethylated SCC patients was found [87]. The methylation of miR-9-3, miR-124-2 and miR-124-3 was individually associated with tumours size of NSCLC patients, independent of age, sex, and smoking habit [88]. Hypermethylation of the promoter region was also found to be responsible for loss of mir-200c in invasive cells [54].

LOH and miRNAs. It was initially shown that miR-128b is a regulator of EGFR in NSCLC cell lines, and that loss of miR-128b is equivalent to loss of tumour suppressor. miR-128b LOH was frequent in tumour samples and correlated significantly with clinical response and survival [89]. MicroRNA miR-101 copy loss is subtype specific event in lung cancer; it is encoded at two loci in the human genome, 1p and 9p. Loss was more frequent at the 9p locus and occurred more often in NSCLC as in small cell lung carcinoma (SCLC). It was suggested that genomic loss of miR-101 may be an early event in NSCLC tumorigenesis, and that DNA deletions likely represents a prominent molecular mechanism of miR-101 down regulation in NSCLC but not in SCLC [90].

Various let-7 genes map to chromosomal regions deleted in human lung cancers. Using NSCLC cell lines, miR-107 and miR-185 were defined as cell cycle regulator miRNAs, localized in frequently altered chromosomal regions in human lung cancer [91].

Table 1. MicroRNAs with known target genes in NSCLC

MicroRNA	Function in NSCLC	Target gene	Studies
let-7g	metastasis	HMGA, KRAS	Park et al., 2010 [60]
miR-7	modulator of EGFR-mediated oncogenesis; proliferation, apoptosis, migration	ERF; Bcl-2	Chou et al., 2010 [57]; Xiong et al., 2011 [58]
miR-15b	induction of cell cycle arrest	Cyclins (D1, D2, E1)	Bandi et al., 2009 [42]; Bandi et al., 2011 [43]
miR-16	induction of cell cycle arrest	Cyclin (D1, D2, E1)	Bandi et al., 2009 [42]; Bandi et al., 2011 [43]
miR-29 family	Epigenetic normalization	DNMT3A, 3B	Fabbri et al., 2007 [84]
miR-30a	EMT, invasion and metastasis	Snai1	Kumarswamy et al., 2012 [55]
miR-34a	proliferation, migration and invasion	Axl	Mudduluru et al., 2011 [39]
miR-17-92 cluster	oncogenic cluster	HIF-1	Taguchi et al., 2008 [45]
miR-93	oncogenes	Fus1	Du et al., 2009 [76]
miR-98	oncogenes	Fus1	Du et al., 2009 [76]
miR-101	proliferation, invasion, apoptosis	EZH2	Zhang et al., 2011 [79]
miR-128b		EGFR	Weiss et al., 2008 [89]
miR-133b	apoptosis	Mcl-1, Bcl2	Crawford et al., 2009 [75]
miR-145	proliferation	c-Myc	Chen et al., 2010 [80]
MicroRNA	Function in NSCLC	Target gene	Studies
miR-197	oncogenes	Fus1	Du et al., 2009 [76]
miR-199a/b	proliferation, migration and invasion	Axl	Mudduluru et al., 2011 [39]
miR-200c	EMT, invasion	TCF8	Hurteau et al., 2007 [53]
miR-210	regulation of mitohondrial function, cell metabolism, survival and modulation of HIF-1 activity	electron transport components	Puissegur et al., 2011 [37]
miR-212	tumour-suppressor, apoptosis; tumour-promoting properties	PED; PTCH1	Incoronato et al, 2010 [77]; Li et al., 2012 [78]
miR-218	suppression and metastasis	PXN	Wu et al., 2010 [68]
miR-328	brain metastases	PRKCA	Arora et al., 2011 [71]
miR-451	survival of tumour cells	RAB14	Wang et al., 2011 [65]

4.1.2. Potential of miRNAs as Biomarkers for Patho-Histological Subtype Classification

Novel chemotherapeutic agents show different efficacy in AD compared with SCC. Therefore accurate classification of NSCLC is clinically important. Precise molecular mechanism that differentiate histopathology, tumour initiation and progression in two major histological subtypes of NSCLC, AD and SCC, are not completely understood [2].

Expression profiling demonstrated differential expression of 6 miRNAs between AD and SCC (miR-205, miR-99b, miR-203, miR-202, miR-102 and miR-204). Separate investigation did not reproduce these findings, but identified larger panel of 34 miRNAs, with most of them up-regulated in lung AD. Furthermore, lineage-specific pattern of miRNA expression was able to distinguish tumours from different types of origin; a group of 48 miRNAs was able to accurately predict the tissue origin of cancer of unknown primary origin in most cases, suggesting the reason for significant differential miRNA expression between lung cancer histological groups or between histologic subtypes within the NSCLC group [2]. In another study, using patients with AD and SCC lung cancer, it was identified that miRNA expression strongly differs between these two entities of NSCLC, particularly in early stages; the differential expressed miRNAs were those located on chromosome loci often altered in lung cancer [92]. Relative quantification of miR-205 and miR-21 was further suggested as promising diagnostic tool, and finally, measurement of miR-205 is suggested as tool for distinction between lung AD and SCC [2]. MicroRNA miR-205 is highly expressed in lung SCC but not in AD, therefore was identified as highly specific markers for SCC, with the assay showing sensitivity of 96 % and specificity of 90 %. There was a very good correlation between the diagnoses established by conventional and miRNA-based methods [93, 94]. However, the relative quantification of miR-205 and miR-21 seems to be a promising diagnostic tool, but is still not completely satisfactory as it may misclassify a non-legible percentage of cases. It cannot be used as substitute but rather as adjunctive diagnostic criterion in selected cases [95]. In trans-thoracic needle aspiration specimens, the let-7 family and miR-205 were quantified. miRNA expression profiles demonstrated considerable, statistically significant difference between lung AD and SCC, showing up-regulation of let-7a/b/c/f/g/i and miR-98 and down-regulation of miR-205 in AD. Profiling of let-7 family and miR-205 is another promising method for differentiating AD from SCC [96].

4.1.3. Potential of miRNAs as Circulating Biomarkers in NSCLC

Using non-invasive diagnostic procedures, the extraction and reliable determination of cell-free miRNAs, circulating in body fluids like plasma, serum, sputum, and others could serve as circulating tumour biomarkers. For lung cancer, it was shown that sufficient miRNAs are present in one millilitre of serum (that are promising prognostic biomarkers), and are significantly increased in plasma of early-stage NSCLC. Serum miRNAs distinguish tumours from normal lung tissues, define histology, growth rate, and clinical outcome. Plasma vesicle-related miRNAs obtained by non-invasive methods could serve as circulating tumour biomarkers of discriminating and prognostic value in NSCLC [97].

Serum miRNAs. Serum miRNAs profiles among different cancer types including NSCLC revealed 28 miRNA missing and 63 new miRNAs detected after the comparison between healthy subjects and lung cancer patients. Using Solexa sequencing serum miRNA expression analysis was investigated in serum for the detection of various cancer and other diseases. The lung cancer specific expression of certain miRNAs was identified in serum; two of them were further validated as NSCLC specific serum miRNAs [98]. Using Solexa sequencing another research was performed; serum miRNA expression analysis was investigated in NSCLC to obtain relevant data for predicting prognosis. Eleven serum miRNAs were found to be altered more than five-fold between longer-survival and shorter-survival groups, and four miRNAs, miR-486, miR-30d, miR-1 and miR-499 were significantly associated with overall survival [99]. Further, miRNA profiling was performed on total RNA extracted from serum obtained from NSCLC patients and controls. The expression of miR-1254 and miR-574-5p was significantly increased in the early-stage NSCLC with respect to the controls [100]. In another study, the expression was measured in serum of lung cancer patients with different histology. The levels of miR-10b, miR-141 and miR-155 were significantly higher in lung cancer patients, including NSCLC patients, than those with benign disease [101]. Furthermore, it was found that cluster of specified miRNAs in peripheral blood may serve as biomarkers for metastatic NSCLC. Serum level of certain miRNAs was assessed in different stages of NSCLC patients compared to control. Statistical significance in serum level was shown for miR-126, miR-183, and miR-222 between advanced NSCLC and controls, but not for miR-

125a-5p, miR-200, and miR-221. MicroRNAs miR-126 and miR-183 were suggested as potential serum biomarkers for metastatic NSCLC [102]. Recently, a test with 80 % accuracy was developed, based on the detection of 34 miRNAs from serum that could identify patients with early stage of NSCLC in a population of asymptomatic high-risk individuals [103].

Plasma miRNAs. Vesicle-related miRNAs in plasma of NSCLC were determinated; five selected miRNAs were validated independently, giving the decrease in expression of let-7f, miR-20b and miR-30e-3p in NSCLC patients. Levels of let-7f and miR-30e-3p distinguished between two groups of patients for stage of disease and possibility of surgery; their levels was associated with short disease-free survival and overall survival, their levels in NSCLC were associated with poor outcome [104]. Aberrant expressions of previously described miRNAs in NSCLC tissue (as associated with early-stage of NSCLC) were further investigated as potential plasma biomarkers for NSCLC. Initial validated expression in paired tumours tissues and plasma were further performed on larger cohort of samples. Of 12 miRNAs, 5 display significant concordance of the expression levels in plasma and the corresponding tumour tissue. Four miRNAs, miR-21, miR-126, miR-210 and miR-486-5p yield 86 % sensitivity and 96 % specificity in distinguishing NSCLC patients from healthy adults. These miRNAs have higher sensitivity in diagnosis of lung AD compared to SCC [105]. In another study, miR-21 was investigated in plasma of NSCLC patients and healthy controls and was significantly higher in NSCLC patients than in age- and sex-matched controls. MicroRNA miR-21 was related to TNM stage, but not related to age, sex, smoking status, histological classification, lymph node status, and metastasis [106]. Further, let-7a miRNA was under-expressed in the blood of NSCLC patients as well as in NSCLC cells and tissues compared to normal control. Authors suggested the possibility of using let-7a miRNA as a serologic marker for lung cancer [107].

Blood cell miRNAs. Using microarray analysis, miRNA expression was also analysed in blood cell samples of patients with NSCLC compared to healthy controls. Using a subset of 24 miRNAs the discrimination between blood cells of NSCLC and healthy individuals was obtained with more than 90 % of accuracy, specificity and sensitivity. This finding support the idea that neoplasia may lead to a deregulation of miRNAs in blood cells of NSCLC patients [108].

Sputum miRNAs. Sputum miRNAs can be used as highly sensitive and specific non-invasive markers for early detection of lung AD, based on expression of miR-21 and miR-155 [109]. For distinguishing lung AD from normal subject, four miRNAs were selected for analysing expression in sputum (miR-21, miR-486, miR-375, and miR-200b) [110].

4.2. snoRNA and NSCLC

Using microarray approach, 6 snoRNAs were recently defined as over-expressed in 22 NSCLC tissue compared with their normal counterparts and those were further examined in plasma [111]. In recent report, emerging evidence suggests that snoRNAs have important roles in tumorigenesis. It was recently shown that SNORA42 was over-expressed in lung tumours, as well as in histological type NSCLC, and as a cause authors suggested genomic amplification. Its expression was inversely correlated with survival of NSCLC. The oncogenic role of SNORA42 activation was proposed [112].

4.3. lncRNA and NSCLC

Using NSCLC cell line, it was already defined, that a novel lncRNA is involved in proliferation arrest. This RNA resides within intron of the HEF1 gene, has no apparent reading frame and may consist of a single large exon. It was named B2 transcript and was proposed to regulate gene expression [113]. Another lncRNA, MALAT-1, is associated with metastasis, but its role in metastatic process remains unknown. Using lung cancer cell lines it was shown that MALAT-1 promotes cell motility through transcriptional and post-transcriptional regulation of motility related gene expression [114].

Other lncRNAs have been also associated with different types of cancers: lincRNA-p21 is implicated in p53 response through the modulation of some p53 dependent gene expression; MEG3 is thought to directly activate the tumour suppressor gene p53; ANRIL is genetically associated with diverse diseases such as diabetes gliomas, coronary diseases, and basal cell carcinomas [25]. It would interest to know whether such scenario is also present in NSCLC.

5. ncRNA and Therapeutic Options

5.1. RNAi and miRNA in Therapeutic Applications

Although it is difficult to introduce long dsRNA strands into mammalian cells due to the interferon response, the use of RNAi as a therapeutic approach has been successful. Among the first applications to reach clinical trials were in the treatment of macular degeneration and respiratory syncytial virus infection, reversal of induced liver failure in mouse models, antiviral therapies, neurodegenerative diseases, and cancer - by silencing up-regulated genes in tumour cells or genes involved in cell division. A key area of research in the use of RNAi for clinical applications is the development of a safe delivery method, which to date has involved mainly viral (lentivirus, adenovirus, adeno-associated virus) and non-viral (nanoparticles, aptamers, stable nucleic-acid-lipid particle) vector systems similar to those suggested for gene therapy [7]. Using RNAi approaches, miRNAs may in future serve as therapeutic targets. For miRNA that is under-expressed, re-introduction of the mature miRNA into the affected tissue would restore the regulation of the target gene. By contrast, over-expressed miRNA could be down regulated by reducing mature miRNA level by its direct targeting [115].

5.2. miRNAs as Therapeutic Targets

Although the pharmacological manipulation of miRNAs is still in its infancy, initial studies have demonstrated that the systemic use of antagomirs is well suited to block miRNA function in small animal models [41]. miRNAs may serve as promising targets of molecular therapy, since inhibition or blockage of their expression should result in increased expression of tumour suppressor genes.

The correlation between the expression of miRNAs and their effects on target oncogenes, on tumorigenesis, and on the proliferation of cancer cells has gained experimental support. MicroRNAs are small molecules, making their *in vivo* delivery feasible. The use of chemically modified oligonucleotides either to target a specific miRNA or disrupt miRNA-mRNA binding may lead to inactivation of pathological miRNA. It has been shown that miRNAs can be delivered systematically, and can reduce invasion, proliferation and growth as well as induce radiosensitivity and resistance. MicroRNAs may therefore serve as therapeutic targets in the future [116].

Replenishing small RNAs. For miRNA that is under-expressed, re-introduction of the mature miRNA into the affected tissue would restore regulation of the target gene. For this purpose, artificial miRNA or the short hairpin duplex, similar to *pre-miRNA*, have been developed to enhance the expression of beneficial miRNAs when introduced into the cell. This suggests that individual miRNAs are potential therapeutic agents and that their expression or delivery can be targeted to appropriate tissue. Most of the developed protocols have used local administration in easily accessible tissue; systemic delivery has also some promising results; the major challenge remains tissue and cell-type specific targeting [116].

Inhibiting small RNAs. ASOs are short and single-stranded antisense oligonucleotides and, in the context of miRNA inhibition, are called AMOs, anti-miRNA oligonucleotides. Over-expressed miRNA can be down-regulated by reducing the mature miRNA level through direct targeting (mature miRNA, *pri-miRNA* or *pre-miRNA*). Chemically engineered oligonucleotides, termed “antagomirs”, have been developed and proven to be efficient and specific silencers of endogenous miRNAs in mice. Chemical modifications and cholesterol conjugations stabilize and facilitate intravenous delivery of antagomirs. They interact with miRNAs in the cytoplasm and lead to specific miRNA down-regulation when injected systemically or locally.

In another approach, miRNA sponges have been developed to inhibit several miRNAs; miRNA sponges possess multiple binding sites and could be useful for sequestering an miRNA family. Furthermore, miR-masks and miR-erasers have also been developed; an miR-mask has been designed for masking the miRNA binding site on target mRNA, whereas an miR-eraser is similar to miR-sponges, except that the miR-eraser uses only two copies of the antisense sequence. Other antisense approaches have been also used to test the possibility of using miRNAs and their corresponding targets as therapeutic targets [116].

Examples for miRNA. Therapeutic delivery was demonstrated using mimics of the tumour suppressor, miR-34a and let-7a, both of which are often down-regulated or lost in lung cancer. It has been shown that re-introduction of let-7 directly represses cancer growth in the lung [117].

Development of therapeutic chemically synthesized miR-34a and lipid-based delivery vehicle block tumour growth in mouse models of NSCLC [118]. Systemic treatment of mouse model of NSCLC led to significant decrease in tumour burden. Mice treated with miR-34a displayed a 60 % reduction in tumour area compared to mice treated with a miRNA control. Similar results were obtained with the let-7 mimic [119]. It was recently shown that a LNA (locked nucleic acid) directed against miR-21 slow down tumour growth in mice [2]. The inhibitory effect of AMOs has been also shown on lung cancer cell lines growth through use of anti-miR-16, anti-miR-21, anti-miR-214, and anti miR-181a [120].

5.3. Targeting Other ncRNAs

Successful inhibition of lncRNAs seems to be more difficult than inhibition of miRNAs. Our growing knowledge of other ncRNAs is also being exploited to develop new therapeutic strategies not only against cancer, but also for other diseased states. The findings regarding lncRNA and Alzheimer disease are attracting the attention of pharmaceutical and biotechnology industries [3].

Conclusion

A lot of efforts have been made in miRNAs as prognostic, diagnostic or therapeutic targets in NSCLC, but there is still a lot of work to do. The rest of ncRNAs, other than miRNAs, in regulation biological functions are more or less unexplored, and this have to be further investigated in future research. Regarding therapeutic approaches, we still need more knowledge concerning which miRNAs to target, how to produce and stabilize them, how to direct them to the tissue. The specificity of drug-like oligonucleotides is important, because of the off-target effect. The off-target effect is also a significant challenge, especially considering that miRNA-mediated repression often requires a homology of only six to seven nucleotides in the seed region of the miRNA and mRNA target site. Toxicity due to chemical modifications, which is used to facilitate cellular uptake and prevent degradation, should be also taken into account.

References

[1] Tong, AW. Small RNAs and non-small cell lung cancer. *Curr. Mol. Med.,* 2006 6, 339-349.

[2] Markou, A; Liang, Y; Lianidou, E. Prognostic, therapeutic and diagnostic potential of microRNAs in non-small cell lung cancer. *Clin. Chem. Lab. Med.,* 2011 49, 1591-1603.

[3] Esteller, M. Non-coding RNAs in human disease. *Nat. Rev. Genet.,* 2011 12, 861-874.

[4] Mattick, JS. The functional genomics of noncoding RNA. *Science,* 2005 309, 1527.

[5] Kaikkonen, MU; Lam, MT; Glass, CK. Non-coding RNAs as regulators of gene expression and epigenetics. *Cardiovasc. Res.,* 2011 90, 430-440.

[6] Zamore, PD; Haley, B. Ribo-gnome: the big world of small RNAs. *Science*, 2005 309, 1519-1524.

[7] Kim, DH; Rossi, JJ. Strategies for silencing human disease using RNA interference. *Nat. Rev. Gen.,* 2007 8, 173-84.

[8] Williams, AE. Functional aspects of animal microRNAs. *Cell Mol. Life Sci.*, 2008 65, 545-562.

[9] Ruvkun, G. Molecular biology. Glimpses of a tiny RNA world. *Science*, 2001 294, 797-9.

[10] Pillai, RS. MicroRNA function: multiple mechanisms for a tiny RNA? *RNA,* 2005 11, 1753-1761.

[11] Bartel, DP. MicroRNAs: genomics, biogenesis, mechanism, and function. *Cell,* 2004 116, 281-297.

[12] Kim, YK; Kim, VN. Processing of intronic microRNAs. *EMBO J,* 2007 26, 775-783.

[13] Pillai, RS; Bhattacharyya, SN; Filipowicz, W. Repression of protein synthesis by miRNAs: how many mechanisms? *Trends Cell Biol.,* 2007 17, 118-126.

[14] Ying, SY; Chang, DC; Lin, SL. The microRNA (miRNA): overview of the RNA genes that modulate gene function. *Mol. Biotechnol.,* 2008 38, 257-68.

[15] Scott, MS; Ono, M. From snoRNA to miRNA: Dual function regulatory non-coding RNAs. *Biochimie,* 2011 93: 1987-92.

[16] Miyoshi, K; Miyoshi, T; Siomi, H. Many ways to generate microRNA-like small RNAs: non-canonical pathways for microRNA production. *Mol. Genet. Genomics,* 2010 284: 95-103.

[17] Perera, RJ; Ray, A. MicroRNAs in the search for understanding human diseases. *BioDrugs,* 2007 21, 97-104.

[18] Holley, CL; Topkara, VK. An introduction to small non-coding RNAs: miRNA and snoRNA *Cardiovasc. Drugs Ther.*, 2011 25, 151-9.

[19] Ioshikhes, I; Roy, S; Sen, CK. Algorithms for mapping of mRNA targets for microRNA. *DNA Cell Biol.,* 2007 26, 265-272.

[20] Kuhn, DE; Martin, MM; Feldman, DS; Terry, AV Jr; Nuovo, GJ; Elton, TS. Experimental validation of miRNA targets. *Methods,* 2008 44, 47-54.

[21] Barnes, MR; Deharo, S; Grocock, RJ; Brown, JR; Sanseau, P. The micro RNA target paradigm: a fundamental and polymorphic control layer of cellular expression. *Expert Opin. Biol. Ther.,* 2007 7, 1387-1399.

[22] Lu, M; Zhang, Q; Deng, M; Miao, J; Guo, Y; Gao, W; Cui, Q. An analysis of human microRNA and disease associations. *PLoS One,* 2008 3, e3420.

[23] Griffiths-Jones, S; Saini, HK; van Dongen, S; Enright, AJ. miRBase: tools for microRNA genomics. *Nucleic Acids Res.,* 2008 36, D154-D158.

[24] Bratkovič, T; Rogelj, B. Biology and applications of small nucleolar RNAs. *Cell Mol. Life Sci.*, 2011 68, 3843-51.

[25] Derrien, T; Guigó, R; Johnson, R. The Long Non-Coding RNAs: A New (P)layer in the "Dark Matter". *Front Genet.,* 2011 2, 107.

[26] Wapinski, O; Chang, HY. Long noncoding RNAs and human disease. *Trends Cell Biol.,* 2011 21, 354-361.

[27] Jay, C; Nemunaitis, J; Chen, P; Fulgham, P; Tong, AW. miRNA profiling for diagnosis and prognosis of human cancer. *DNA Cell Biol.,* 2007 26, 293-300.

[28] Blenkiron, C; Miska, EA. miRNAs in cancer: approaches, aetiology, diagnostics and therapy. *Hum. Mol. Genet.,* 2007 16, R106-13.

[29] Zhang, B; Pan ,X; Cobb, GP; Anderson, TA. microRNAs as oncogenes and tumor suppressors. *Dev. Biol.,* 2007 302, 1-12.

[30] Kosaka, N; Iguchi, H; Ochiya, T. Circulating microRNA in body fluid: a new potential biomarker for cancer diagnosis and prognosis.*Cancer Sci.,* 2010 101, 2087-92.

[31] Cho, WC. MicroRNAs: potential biomarkers for cancer diagnosis, prognosis and targets for therapy. *Int. J. Biochem. Cell Biol.,* 2010 42, 1273-81.

[32] Kao, S; Shiau, CK; Gu, DL; Ho, CM; Su, WH; Chen, CF; Lin, CH; Jou, YS. IGDB.NSCLC: integrated genomic database of non-small cell lung cancer. *Nucleic Acids Res.*, 2012 40, D972-7.

[33] Karube, Y; Tanaka, H; Osada, H; Tomida, S; Tatematsu, Y; Yanagisawa, K; Yatabe, Y; Takamizawa, J; Miyoshi, S; Mitsudomi, T; Takahashi, T. Reduced expression of Dicer associated with poor prognosis in lung cancer patients. *Cancer Sci.*, 2005 96, 111-5.

[34] Chiosea, S; Jelezcova, E; Chandran, U; Luo, J; Mantha, G; Sobol, RW; Dacic, S. Overexpression of Dicer in precursor lesions of lung adenocarcinoma. *Cancer Res.*, 2007 67, 2345-50.

[35] Kulshreshtha, R; Ferracin, M; Negrini, M; Calin, GA; Davuluri, RV; Ivan, M. Regulation of microRNA expression: the hypoxic component. *Cell Cycle*, 2007 6, 1426-31.

[36] Kulshreshtha, R; Davuluri, RV; Calin, GA; Ivan, M. A microRNA component of the hypoxic response. *Cell Death Differ.*, 2008 15, 667-71.

[37] Puisségur, MP; Mazure, NM; Bertero, T; Pradelli, L; Grosso, S; Robbe-Sermesant, K; Maurin, T; Lebrigand, K; Cardinaud, B; Hofman, V; Fourre, S; Magnone, V; Ricci, JE; Pouysségur, J; Gounon, P; Hofman, P; Barbry, P; Mari, B. miR-210 is overexpressed in late stages of lung cancer and mediates mitochondrial alterations associated with modulation of HIF-1 activity. *Cell Death Differ.*, 2011 18, 465-78.

[38] Gallardo, E; Navarro, A; Viñolas, N; Marrades, RM; Diaz, T; Gel, B; Quera, A; Bandres, E; Garcia-Foncillas, J; Ramirez, J; Monzo, M. miR-34a as a prognostic marker of relapse in surgically resected non-small-cell lung cancer. *Carcinogenesis*, 2009 30, 1903-9.

[39] Mudduluru, G; Ceppi, P; Kumarswamy, R; Scagliotti, GV; Papotti, M; Allgayer H. Regulation of Axl receptor tyrosine kinase expression by miR-34a and miR-199a/b in solid cancer. *Oncogene,* 2011 30, 2888-99.

[40] Donnem, T; Fenton, CG; Lonvik, K; Berg, T; Eklo, K; Andersen, S; Stenvold, H; Al-Shibli, K; Al-Saad, S; Bremnes, RM; Busund, LT. MicroRNA Signatures in Tumor Tissue Related to Angiogenesis in Non-Small Cell Lung Cancer. *PLoS One*, 2012 7, e29671.

[41] Kuehbacher, A; Urbich, C; Dimmeler, S. Targeting microRNA expression to regulate angiogenesis. *Trends Pharmacol. Sci.*, 2008 29, 12-5.

[42] Bandi, N; Zbinden, S; Gugger, M; Arnold, M; Kocher, V; Hasan, L; Kappeler, A; Brunner, T; Vassella, E. miR-15a and miR-16 are implicated in cell cycle regulation in a Rb-dependent manner and are frequently deleted or down-regulated in non-small cell lung cancer. *Cancer Res.*, 2009 69, 5553-9.

[43] Bandi, N; Vassella, E. miR-34a and miR-15a/16 are co-regulated in non-small cell lung cancer and control cell cycle progression in a synergistic and Rb-dependent manner. *Mol. Cancer*, 2011 10, 55.

[44] Navarro, A; Diaz, T; Gallardo, E; Viñolas, N; Marrades, RM; Gel, B; Campayo, M; Quera, A; Bandres, E; Garcia-Foncillas, J; Ramirez, J; Monzo, M. Prognostic implications of miR-16 expression levels in resected non-small-cell lung cancer. *J. Surg. Oncol.*, 2011 103, 411-5.

[45] Taguchi, A; Yanagisawa, K; Tanaka, M; Cao, K; Matsuyama, Y; Goto, H; Takahashi, T. Identification of hypoxia-inducible factor-1 alpha as a novel target for miR-17-92 microRNA cluster. *Cancer Res.*, 2008 68, 5540-5.

[46] Crawford, M; Brawner, E; Batte, K; Yu, L; Hunter, MG; Otterson, GA; Nuovo, G; Marsh, CB; Nana-Sinkam, SP. MicroRNA-126 inhibits invasion in non-small cell lung carcinoma cell lines. *Biochem. Biophys. Res. Commun.*, 2008 373, 607-12.

[47] Donnem, T; Lonvik, K; Eklo, K; Berg, T; Sorbye, SW; Al-Shibli, K; Al-Saad, S; Andersen, S; Stenvold, H; Bremnes, RM; Busund, LT. Independent and tissue-specific prognostic impact of miR-126 in nonsmall cell lung cancer: coexpression with vascular endothelial growth factor-A predicts poor survival. *Cancer*, 2011 117, 3193-200.

[48] Ma, X; Becker Buscaglia, LE; Barker, JR; Li, Y. MicroRNAs in NF-kB signaling. *J. Mol. Cell Biol.*, 2011 3, 159-66.

[49] Williams, AE; Perry, MM; Moschos, SA; Larner-Svensson, HM; Lindsay, MA. Role of miRNA-146a in the regulation of the innate immune response and cancer. *Biochem. Soc. Trans.*, 2008 36, 1211-5.

[50] Li, L; Chen, XP; Li, YJ. MicroRNA-146a and human disease. *Scand. J. Immunol.*, 2010 71, 227-31.

[51] Patnaik, SK; Kannisto, E; Mallick, R; Yendamuri, S. Overexpression of the lung cancer-prognostic miR-146b microRNAs has a minimal and negative effect on the malignant phenotype of A549 lung cancer cells. *PLoS One*, 2011 6, e22379.

[52] Donnem, T; Eklo, K; Berg, T; Sorbye, SW; Lonvik, K; Al-Saad, S; Al-Shibli, K; Andersen, S; Stenvold, H; Bremnes, RM; Busund, LT. Prognostic impact of MiR-155 in non-small cell lung cancer evaluated by in situ hybridization. *J. Transl. Med.*, 2011 9, 6.

[53] Hurteau, GJ; Carlson, JA; Spivack, SD; Brock, GJ. Overexpression of the microRNA hsa-miR-200c leads to reduced expression of transcription factor 8 and increased expression of E-cadherin. *Cancer Res.*, 2007 67, 7972-6.

[54] Ceppi, P; Mudduluru, G; Kumarswamy, R; Rapa, I; Scagliotti, GV; Papotti, M; Allgayer, H. Loss of miR-200c expression induces an aggressive, invasive, and chemoresistant phenotype in non-small cell lung cancer. *Mol. Cancer Res.*, 2010 8, 1207-16.

[55] Kumarswamy, R; Mudduluru, G; Ceppi, P; Muppala, S; Kozlowski, M; Niklinski, J; Papotti, M; Allgayer, H. MicroRNA-30a inhibits epithelial-to-mesenchymal transition by targeting Snai1 and is downregulated in non-small cell lung cancer. *Int. J. Cancer*, 2012 130, 2044-53.

[56] Cho, WC; Chow, AS; Au, JS. Restoration of tumour suppressor hsa-miR-145 inhibits cancer cell growth in lung adenocarcinoma patients with epidermal growth factor receptor mutation. *Eur. J. Cancer*, 2009 45, 2197-206.

[57] Chou, YT; Lin, HH; Lien, YC; Wang, YH; Hong, CF; Kao, YR; Lin, SC; Chang, YC; Lin, SY; Chen, SJ; Chen, HC; Yeh, SD; Wu, CW. EGFR promotes lung tumorigenesis by activating miR-7 through a Ras/ERK/Myc pathway that targets the Ets2 transcriptional repressor ERF. *Cancer Res.*, 2010 70, 8822-31.

[58] Xiong, S; Zheng, Y; Jiang, P; Liu, R; Liu, X; Chu, Y. MicroRNA-7 inhibits the growth of human non-small cell lung cancer A549 cells through targeting BCL-2. *Int. J. Biol. Sci.*, 2011 7, 805-14.

[59] Takamizawa, J; Konishi, H; Yanagisawa, K; Tomida, S; Osada, H; Endoh, H; Harano, T; Yatabe, Y; Nagino, M; Nimura, Y; Mitsudomi, T; Takahashi, T. Reduced expression of the let-7 microRNAs in human lung cancers in association with shortened postoperative survival. *Cancer Res.*, 2004 64, 3753-6.

[60] Park, S; Minai-Tehrani, A; Xu, CX; Chang, SH; Woo, MA; Noh, MS; Lee, ES; Lim, HT; An, GH; Lee, KH; Sung, HJ; Beck, GR; Cho, MH. Suppression of A549 lung cancer cell migration by precursor let-7g microRNA. *Mol. Med. Report*, 2010 3, 1007-13.

[61] Zhang, JG; Wang, JJ; Zhao, F; Liu, Q; Jiang, K; Yang, GH. MicroRNA-21 (miR-21) represses tumor suppressor PTEN and promotes growth and invasion in non-small cell lung cancer (NSCLC). *Clin. Chim. Acta*, 2010 411, 846-52.

[62] Seike, M; Goto, A; Okano, T; Bowman, ED; Schetter, AJ; Horikawa, I; Mathe, EA; Jen, J; Yang, P; Sugimura, H; Gemma, A; Kudoh, S; Croce, CM; Harris, CC. MiR-21 is an EGFR-regulated anti-apoptotic factor in lung cancer in never-smokers. *Proc. Natl. Acad. Sci. U S A*, 2009 106, 12085-90.

[63] Hatley, ME; Patrick, DM; Garcia, MR; Richardson, JA; Bassel-Duby, R; van Rooij, E; Olson, EN. Modulation of K-Ras-dependent lung tumorigenesis by MicroRNA-21. *Cancer Cell*, 2010 18, 282-93.

[64] Wang, XC; Tian, LL; Jiang, XY; Wang, YY; Li, DG; She, Y; Chang, JH; Meng, AM. The expression and function of miRNA-451 in non-small cell lung cancer. *Cancer Lett.*, 2011 311, 203-9.

[65] Wang, R; Wang, ZX; Yang, JS; Pan, X; De, W; Chen, LB. MicroRNA-451 functions as a tumor suppressor in human non-small cell lung cancer by targeting ras-related protein 14 (RAB14). *Oncogene*, 2011 30, 2644-58.

[66] Wang, XC; Tian, LL; Wu, HL; Jiang, XY; Du, LQ; Zhang, H; Wang, YY; Wu, HY; Li, DG; She, Y; Liu, QF; Fan, FY; Meng, AM. Expression of miRNA-130a in nonsmall cell lung cancer. *Am. J. Med. Sci.*, 2010 340, 385-8.

[67] Davidson, MR; Larsen, JE; Yang, IA; Hayward, NK; Clarke, BE; Duhig, EE; Passmore, LH; Bowman, RV; Fong, KM. MicroRNA-218 is deleted and downregulated in lung squamous cell carcinoma. *PLoS One*, 2010 5, e12560.

[68] Wu, DW; Cheng, YW; Wang, J; Chen, CY; Lee, H. Paxillin predicts survival and relapse in non-small cell lung cancer by microRNA-218 targeting. *Cancer Res.*, 2010 70, 10392-401.

[69] Jiang, L; Huang, Q; Zhang, S; Zhang, Q; Chang, J; Qiu, X; Wang, E. Hsa-miR-125a-3p and hsa-miR-125a-5p are downregulated in non-small cell lung cancer and have inverse effects on invasion and migration of lung cancer cells. *BMC Cancer*, 2010 10, 318.

[70] Wang, X; Ling, C; Bai, Y; Zhao, J. MicroRNA-206 is associated with invasion and metastasis of lung cancer. *Anat. Rec. (Hoboken)*, 2011 294, 88-92.

[71] Arora, S; Ranade, AR; Tran, NL; Nasser, S; Sridhar, S; Korn, RL; Ross, JT; Dhruv, H; Foss, KM; Sibenaller, Z; Ryken, T; Gotway, MB; Kim, S; Weiss, GJ. MicroRNA-328 is associated with (non-small) cell lung cancer (NSCLC) brain metastasis and mediates NSCLC migration. *Int. J. Cancer*, 2011 129, 2621-31.

[72] Chen, LT; Xu, SD; Xu, H; Zhang, JF; Ning, JF; Wang, SF. MicroRNA-378 is associated with non-small cell lung cancer brain metastasis by promoting cell migration, invasion and tumor angiogenesis. *Med. Oncol.*, 2012 29, 1673-80.

[73] Võsa, U; Vooder, T; Kolde, R; Fischer, K; Välk, K; Tõnisson, N; Roosipuu, R; Vilo, J; Metspalu, A; Annilo, T. Identification of miR-374a as a prognostic marker for survival in patients with early-stage nonsmall cell lung cancer. *Genes Chromosomes Cancer*, 2011 50, 812-22.

[74] Gao W; Yu Y; Cao H; Shen H; Li X; Pan S; Shu Y. Deregulated expression of miR-21, miR-143 and miR-181a in non small cell lung cancer is related to clinicopathologic characteristics or patient prognosis. *Biomed. Pharmacother.*, 2010 64, 399-408.

[75] Crawford M; Batte K; Yu L; Wu X; Nuovo GJ; Marsh CB; Otterson GA; Nana-Sinkam SP. MicroRNA 133B targets pro-survival molecules MCL-1 and BCL2L2 in lung cancer. *Biochem. Biophys. Res. Commun.*, 2009 388, 483-9.

[76] Du L; Schageman JJ; Subauste MC; Saber B; Hammond SM; Prudkin L; Wistuba II; Ji L; Roth JA; Minna JD; Pertsemlidis A. miR-93, miR-98, and miR-197 regulate expression of tumor suppressor gene FUS1. *Mol. Cancer Res.*, 2009 7,1234-43.

[77] Incoronato, M; Garofalo, M; Urso, L; Romano, G; Quintavalle, C; Zanca, C; Iaboni, M; Nuovo, G; Croce, CM; Condorelli, G. miR-212 increases tumor necrosis factor-related apoptosis-inducing ligand sensitivity in non-small cell lung cancer by targeting the antiapoptotic protein PED. *Cancer Res.*, 2010 70, 3638-46.

[78] Li, Y; Zhang, D; Chen, C; Ruan, Z; Li, Y; Huang, Y. MiR-212 displays Tumor Promoting properties in NSCLC Cells and targets the Hedgehog Pathway Receptor PTCH1. *Mol. Biol. Cell,* 2012 23, 1423-34.

[79] Zhang, JG; Guo, JF; Liu, DL; Liu, Q; Wang, JJ. MicroRNA-101 exerts tumor-suppressive functions in non-small cell lung cancer through directly targeting enhancer of zeste homolog 2. *J. Thorac. Oncol.*, 2011 6, 671-8.

[80] Chen, Z; Zeng, H; Guo, Y; Liu, P; Pan, H; Deng, A; Hu, J. miRNA-145 inhibits non-small cell lung cancer cell proliferation by targeting c-Myc. *J. Exp. Clin. Cancer Res.*, 2010 29, 151.

[81] Chin, LJ; Ratner, E; Leng, S; Zhai, R; Nallur, S; Babar, I; Muller, RU; Straka, E; Su, L; Burki, EA; Crowell, RE; Patel, R; Kulkarni, T; Homer, R; Zelterman, D; Kidd, KK; Zhu, Y; Christiani, DC; Belinsky, SA; Slack, FJ; Weidhaas, JB. A SNP in a let-7 microRNA complementary site in the KRAS 3' untranslated region increases non-small cell lung cancer risk. *Cancer Res.*, 2008 68, 8535-40.

[82] Hu, Z; Chen, J; Tian, T; Zhou, X; Gu, H; Xu, L; Zeng, Y; Miao, R; Jin, G; Ma, H; Chen, Y; Shen, H. Genetic variants of miRNA sequences and non-small cell lung cancer survival. *J. Clin. Invest.*, 2008 118, 2600-8.

[83] Hu, Z; Shu, Y; Chen, Y; Chen, J; Dong, J; Liu, Y; Pan, S; Xu, L; Xu, J; Wang, Y; Dai, J; Ma, H; Jin, G; Shen, H. Genetic polymorphisms in the precursor MicroRNA flanking region and non-small cell lung cancer survival. *Am. J. Respir. Crit. Care Med.*, 2011 183, 641-8.

[84] Fabbri, M; Garzon, R; Cimmino, A; Liu, Z; Zanesi, N; Callegari, E; Liu, S; Alder, H; Costinean, S; Fernandez-Cymering, C; Volinia, S; Guler, G; Morrison, CD; Chan, KK; Marcucci, G; Calin, GA; Huebner, K; Croce, CM. MicroRNA-29 family reverts aberrant methylation in lung cancer by targeting DNA methyltransferases 3A and 3B. *Proc. Natl. Acad. Sci. U S A*, 2007 104, 15805-10.

[85] Brueckner, B; Stresemann, C; Kuner, R; Mund, C; Musch, T; Meister, M; Sültmann, H; Lyko, F. The human let-7a-3 locus contains an epigenetically regulated microRNA gene with oncogenic function. *Cancer Res.*, 2007 67, 1419-23.

[86] Wang, Z; Chen, Z; Gao, Y; Li, N; Li, B; Tan, F; Tan, X; Lu, N; Sun, Y; Sun, J; Sun, N; He, J. DNA hypermethylation of microRNA-34b/c has prognostic value for stage I non-small cell lung cancer. *Cancer Biol. Ther.*, 2011 11, 490-6.

[87] Heller, G; Weinzierl, M; Noll, C; Babinsky, V; Ziegler, B; Altenberger, C; Minichsdorfer, C; Lang, G; Dome, B; End-Pfutzenreuter, A; Arns, BM; Grin, Y; Klepetko, W; Zielinski, CC; Zochbauer-Muller, S.Genome-wide microRNA expression profiling identifies miR-9-3 and miR-193a as targets for DNA methylation in non-small cell lung cancers. *Clin. Cancer Res.*, 2012 18, 1619-29.

[88] Kitano, K; Watanabe, K; Emoto, N; Kage, H; Hamano, E; Nagase, T; Sano, A; Murakawa, T; Nakajima, J; Goto, A; Fukayama, M; Yatomi, Y; Ohishi, N; Takai, D. CpG island methylation of microRNAs is associated with tumor size and recurrence of non-small-cell lung cancer. *Cancer Sci.*, 2011 102, 2126-31.

[89] Weiss, GJ; Bemis, LT; Nakajima, E; Sugita, M; Birks, DK; Robinson, WA; Varella-Garcia, M; Bunn, PA Jr; Haney, J; Helfrich, BA; Kato, H; Hirsch, FR; Franklin, WA. EGFR regulation by microRNA in lung cancer: correlation with clinical response and survival to gefitinib and EGFR expression in cell lines. *Ann. Oncol.*, 2008 19,1053-9.

[90] Thu, KL; Chari, R; Lockwood, WW; Lam, S; Lam, WL. miR-101 DNA copy loss is a prominent subtype specific event in lung cancer. *J. Thorac. Oncol.*, 2011 6, 1594-8.

[91] Takahashi, Y; Forrest, AR; Maeno, E; Hashimoto, T; Daub, CO; Yasuda, J. MiR-107 and MiR-185 can induce cell cycle arrest in human non small cell lung cancer cell lines. *PLoS One*, 2009 4, e6677.

[92] Landi, MT; Zhao, Y; Rotunno, M; Koshiol, J; Liu, H; Bergen, AW; Rubagotti, M; Goldstein, AM; Linnoila, I; Marincola, FM; Tucker, MA; Bertazzi, PA; Pesatori, AC; Caporaso, NE; McShane, LM; Wang, E. MicroRNA expression differentiates histology and predicts survival of lung cancer. *Clin Cancer Res.*, 2010 16, 430-41.

[93] Bishop, JA; Benjamin, H; Cholakh, H; Chajut, A; Clark, DP; Westra, WH. Accurate classification of non-small cell lung carcinoma using a novel microRNA-based approach. *Clin. Cancer Res.*, 2010 16, 610-9.

[94] Lebanony, D; Benjamin, H; Gilad, S; Ezagouri, M; Dov, A; Ashkenazi, K; Gefen, N; Izraeli, S; Rechavi, G; Pass, H; Nonaka, D; Li, J; Spector, Y; Rosenfeld, N; Chajut, A; Cohen, D; Aharonov, R; Mansukhani, M. Diagnostic assay based on hsa-miR-205 expression distinguishes squamous from nonsquamous non-small-cell lung carcinoma. *J. Clin. Oncol.*, 2009 27, 2030-7.

[95] Del Vescovo, V; Cantaloni, C; Cucino, A; Girlando, S; Silvestri, M; Bragantini, E; Fasanella, S; Cuorvo, LV; Palma, PD; Rossi, G; Papotti, M; Pelosi, G; Graziano, P; Cavazza, A; Denti, MA; Barbareschi, M. miR-205 Expression levels in nonsmall cell lung cancer do not always distinguish adenocarcinomas from squamous cell carcinomas. *Am. J. Surg. Pathol.*, 2011 35, 268-75.

[96] Fassina, A; Cappellesso, R; Fassan, M. Classification of non-small cell lung carcinoma in transthoracic needle specimens using microRNA expression profiling. *Chest*, 2011 140, 1305-11.

[97] Gao, W; Liu, L; Lu, X; Shu, Y. Circulating microRNAs: possible prediction biomarkers for personalized therapy of non-small-cell lung carcinoma. *Clin. Lung Cancer*, 2011 12, 14-7.

[98] Chen, X; Ba, Y; Ma, L; Cai, X; Yin, Y; Wang, K; Guo, J; Zhang, Y; Chen, J; Guo, X; Li, Q; Li, X; Wang, W; Zhang, Y; Wang, J; Jiang, X; Xiang, Y; Xu, C; Zheng, P; Zhang, J; Li, R; Zhang, H; Shang, X; Gong, T; Ning, G; Wang, J; Zen, K; Zhang, J; Zhang, CY. Characterization of microRNAs in serum: a novel class of biomarkers for diagnosis of cancer and other diseases. *Cell Res.*, 2008 18, 997-1006.

[99] Hu, Z; Chen, X; Zhao, Y; Tian, T; Jin, G; Shu, Y; Chen, Y; Xu, L; Zen, K; Zhang, C; Shen, H. Serum microRNA signatures identified in a genome-wide serum microRNA expression profiling predict survival of non-small-cell lung cancer. *J. Clin. Oncol.*, 2010 28, 1721-6.

[100] Foss, KM; Sima, C; Ugolini, D; Neri, M; Allen, KE; Weiss, GJ. miR-1254 and miR-574-5p: serum-based microRNA biomarkers for early-stage non-small cell lung cancer. *J. Thorac. Oncol.*, 2011 6, 482-8.

[101] Roth, C; Kasimir-Bauer, S; Pantel, K; Schwarzenbach, H. Screening for circulating nucleic acids and caspase activity in the peripheral blood as potential diagnostic tools in lung cancer. *Mol. Oncol.*, 2011 5, 281-91.

[102] Lin, Q; Mao, W; Shu, Y; Lin, F; Liu, S; Shen, H; Gao, W; Li, S; Shen, D. A cluster of specified microRNAs in peripheral blood as biomarkers for metastatic non-small-cell lung cancer by stem-loop RT-PCR. *J. Cancer Res. Clin. Oncol.*, 2012 138, 85-93.

[103] Bianchi, F; Nicassio, F; Marzi, M; Belloni, E; Dall'olio, V; Bernard, L; Pelosi, G; Maisonneuve, P; Veronesi, G; Di Fiore, PP. A serum circulating miRNA diagnostic test to identify asymptomatic high-risk individuals with early stage lung cancer. *EMBO Mol. Med.*, 2011 3, 495-503.

[104] Silva, J; García, V; Zaballos, Á; Provencio, M; Lombardía, L; Almonacid, L; García, JM; Domínguez, G; Peña, C; Diaz, R; Herrera, M; Varela, A; Bonilla, F. Vesicle-related microRNAs in plasma of nonsmall cell lung cancer patients and correlation with survival. *Eur. Respir. J.*, 2011 37, 617-23.

[105] Shen, J; Todd, NW; Zhang, H; Yu, L; Lingxiao, X; Mei, Y; Guarnera, M; Liao, J; Chou, A; Lu, CL; Jiang, Z; Fang, H; Katz, RL; Jiang, F. Plasma microRNAs as potential biomarkers for non-small-cell lung cancer. *Lab. Invest.*, 2011 91, 579-87.

[106] Wei, J; Gao, W; Zhu, CJ; Liu, YQ; Mei, Z; Cheng, T; Shu, YQ. Identification of plasma microRNA-21 as a biomarker for early detection and chemosensitivity of non-small cell lung cancer. *Chin. J. Cancer*, 2011 30, 407-14.

[107] Jeong, HC; Kim, EK; Lee, JH; Lee, JM; Yoo, HN; Kim, JK. Aberrant expression of let-7a miRNA in the blood of non-small cell lung cancer patients. *Mol. Med. Report*, 2011 4, 383-7.

[108] Keller, A; Leidinger, P; Borries, A; Wendschlag, A; Wucherpfennig, F; Scheffler, M; Huwer, H; Lenhof, HP; Meese, E. miRNAs in lung cancer - studying complex fingerprints in patient's blood cells by microarray experiments. *BMC Cancer*, 2009 9, 353.

[109] Xie, Y; Todd, NW; Liu, Z; Zhan, M; Fang, H; Peng, H; Alattar, M; Deepak, J; Stass, SA; Jiang, F. Altered miRNA expression in sputum for diagnosis of non-small cell lung cancer. *Lung Cancer*, 2010 67, 170-6.

[110] Yu, L; Todd, NW; Xing, L; Xie, Y; Zhang, H; Liu, Z; Fang, H; Zhang, J; Katz, RL; Jiang, F. Early detection of lung adenocarcinoma in sputum by a panel of microRNA markers. *Int. J. Cancer*, 2010 127, 2870-8.

[111] Liao, J; Yu, L; Mei, Y; Guarnera, M; Shen, J; Li, R; Liu, Z; Jiang, F. Small nucleolar RNA signatures as biomarkers for non-small-cell lung cancer. *Mol. Cancer*, 2010 9, 198.

[112] Mei, YP; Liao, JP; Shen, JP; Yu, L; Liu, BL; Liu, L; Li, RY; Ji, L; Dorsey, SG; Jiang, ZR; Katz, RL; Wang, JY; Jiang, F. Small nucleolar RNA 42 acts as an oncogene in lung tumorigenesis. *Oncogene*, 2012 31, 2794-804.

[113] Jacquot, C; Carbonnelle, D; Tomasoni, C; Papaconstadinou, A; Roussis, V; Roussakis, C. Identification of a novel putative non-coding RNA involved in proliferation arrest of a non-small cell lung carcinoma cell line treated with an original chemical substance, methyl-4-methoxy-3-(3-methyl-2-butanoyl) benzoate. *Int. J. Oncol.*, 2004 25, 519-27.

[114] Tano, K; Mizuno, R; Okada, T; Rakwal, R; Shibato, J; Masuo, Y; Ijiri, K; Akimitsu, N. MALAT-1 enhances cell motility of lung adenocarcinoma cells by influencing the expression of motility-related genes. *FEBS Lett.*, 2010 584, 4575-80.

[115] Soifer, HS; Rossi, JJ; Saetrom, P. MicroRNA in disease and potential therapeutic applications. *Mol. Ther.,* 2007 15, 2070-9.

[116] van Rooij, E. The art of microRNA research. *Circ. Res.,* 2011 108, 219-34.

[117] Kumar, MS; Erkeland, SJ; Pester, RE; Chen, CY; Ebert, MS; Sharp, PA; Jacks, T. Suppression of non-small cell lung tumor development by the let-7 microRNA family. *Proc. Natl. Acad. Sci. U S A*, 2008 105, 3903-8.

[118] Wiggins, JF; Ruffino, L; Kelnar, K; Omotola, M; Patrawala, L; Brown, D; Bader, AG. Development of a lung cancer therapeutic based on the tumor suppressor microRNA-34. *Cancer Res.*, 2010 70, 5923-30.

[119] Trang, P; Wiggins, JF; Daige, CL; Cho, C; Omotola, M; Brown, D; Weidhaas, JB; Bader, AG; Slack, FJ. Systemic delivery of tumor suppressor microRNA mimics using a neutral lipid emulsion inhibits lung tumors in mice. *Mol. Ther.*, 2011 19, 1116-22.

[120] Fei, J; Lan, F; Guo, M; Li, Y; Liu, Y. Inhibitory effects of anti-miRNA oligonucleotides (AMOs) on A549 cell growth. *J. Drug Target*, 2008 16, 688-93.

In: Non-Small Cell Lung Cancer: New Research
Editor: Lina Pasquariello
ISBN: 978-1-62417-804-7

Chapter 3

Epigenetics in Lung Cancer: Preclinical and Clinical Advances

Benjamin F. Chu and Gregory A. Otterson*
Department of Medicine, Division of Medical Oncology; The Ohio State University Comprehensive Cancer Center and Solove Research Institute, Columbus, OH, US

Abstract

Lung cancer is the leading cause of cancer death in the United States and worldwide. Treatment strategies and options have expanded greatly in recent years, including the use of molecular targeted agents. Targeted therapies, exploiting cancer specific genetic "driver" mutations, while very powerful, are unfortunately limited to subsets of the overall population. In this chapter, we will review recent developments of novel therapeutic approach through epigenetic alteration. Epigenetic modification was first discovered by understanding inherited imprinting disorders. Since the discovery of the role of epigenetics in cancer, major strides in deciphering the biology of epigenetic machinery have been made, including DNA methylation, histone acetylation and dynamic alteration of nucleosomal remodeling during the cell cycle. These changes occur early during tumorigenesis as seen in many solid tumors. Biomarkers utilizing abnormal epigenetic signatures are being evaluated for early cancer detection of preneoplastic and preinvasive lesions. In addition, since epigenetic alterations are potentially reversible, as opposed to irreversible genetic alterations (such as insertions, deletions, point mutations and translocations), they offer potential targets for cancer therapy. Epigenetic modulations through DNA methylation and histone deacetylase (HDAC) inhibitors are only beginning to be explored in the clinical setting. Given the almost universal finding of epigenetic alterations in lung cancer, translation of basic epigenomic research into the development of novel agents will provide a new perspective for lung cancer treatments.

Keywords: Methylation, histone acetylation, cancer stem cell, microRNA, epigenetics, epigenomics, HDAC, DNMT, lung cancer

* E-mail: greg.otterson@osumc.edu., Tel.: (614) 293-9424., Fax: (614) 293-7529.

Introduction

More than 200,000 patients are diagnosed with lung cancer in the United States every year and more than 150,000 of these patients eventually die from their diagnosis[1]. Lung cancer accounts for approximately 14% of cancer diagnoses behind prostate and breast cancer in both genders; however, it remains the leading cause of death in the United States for both men and women[1]. Cigarette smoking is historically the most common etiologic agent of lung cancer, though additional lung carcinogens have been identified including asbestos, radon, second hand smoke and others.

Cancer cells have numerous genetic mutations. The list of genes associated with the transformed cancer cell has grown dramatically since the completion of Human Genome project. Overlying the catalogue of genes altered in the cancer genome however, there are processes of modifying the environment of gene transcription and translation during cancer development. Regulation of the transcriptional and translational environment has proven to be an important biologic mechanism controlling cellular differentiation, proliferation, apoptosis, genetic silencing/imprinting, cell aging and cancer development.

This process, referred to as epigenetic, is defined by a heritable characteristic that is passed on to daughter cells without involving modification of primary nucleotide sequence[2]. Its heritability allows propagation of epigenetic modifications, analogous to the heritability of genetic mutations accumulating in precancerous cells, eventually leading to the cancer phenotype.

Understanding the mechanism of epigenetic regulation will provide an invaluable insight for a complex biological network of dysregulation in cancer cells [3].

Epigenetic Biology

One of the most intensively studied epigenetic changes is DNA methylation. Methylation occurs preferentially at cytosines within the context of a subsequent guanosine residue (a CpG dinucleotide). Methylation of cytosine residues can happen throughout the genome, and involves the addition of a one carbon methyl group to the 5 position of cytosine. This "extra-nucleotide" modification is catalyzed by enzymes called DNA methyltransferase proteins (DNMTs).

There are two "de novo" methyltransferases (DNMT3a and DNMT3b) and one "maintenance" methyltransferase (DNMT1) responsible for establishing and maintaining a pattern of DNA methylation and influencing gene expression.

CpG dinucleotides are not evenly distributed throughout the genome [4,5]. It has been postulated that DNA methylation may promote CpG dinucleotide depletion during evolution, leaving small clusters of CpG rich regions. These regions, termed CpG islands, are areas of at least 200 base pairs of DNA with a greater than expected GC content and a relative preponderance of C followed by G. CpG islands are associated with promoter elements in as much as 60% of human genes [6]. In normal cells, CpG islands are hypomethylated to allow transcription of genes controlled by the promoters.

Areas that contain CpG dinucleotides but do not meet the criteria for CpG islands, are typically heavily methylated in normal cells. Interestingly, this pattern of methylation is reversed in cancer cell where CpG islands tend to become hypermethylated, while the scattered CpG dinucleotides (non CpG islands) outside of the promoter regions are relatively hypomethylated [7,8]. This finding initially generated a somewhat confusing conundrum as both hypo- and hyper- methylated areas in cancer cells were described. It later become clear that promoter region hypermethylation in CpG islands suppresses downstream genes while larger scale global hypomethylation has the tendency to promote chromosomal instability commonly seen in precancerous cells.

DNA Hypomethylation

The first epigenetic abnormality observed in cancer cells was DNA hypomethylation in small cell lung cancer[7]. Hypomethylation has indeed been an important feature of cancer development through transcriptionally awakening a normally inert gene. Cancer-testis antigens (CTA) are immunogenic proteins that are usually suppressed outside of germinal cell lines. The regulation of these proteins has been under intensive investigation because numerous CTA's, such as NY-ESO-1, MAGE-A1, and MAGE-A3, are reactivated in many malignancies, including lung cancers. A recent study using microarray data of lung carcinoma tissues showed that CTA gene groups are among the most highly expressed genes in lung cancer cells. Within the known CTA gene family, 90% are expressed in squamous carcinoma, 62% in bronchioalveolar and 67% in adenocarcinoma [9]. Suppression of these genes in lung cancer cell lines coincided with recruitment of methylation machinery in the promoter regions as well as increased DNA methylation while expression of CTA's is associated with DNA demethylation [10,11]. Deciphering the mechanism of regulation for CTA expression is, therefore, of great interest. An interacting partner of CTA's, Brother of the Regulator of Imprinted Sites (BORIS), which was first discovered as a key transcriptional factor in imprinting mechanism, may play a central role in regulating MAGE gene family demethylation processes in both NSCLC and SCLC cell lines [12]. More interestingly, CCCTC-binding factor (CTCF), a paralogous regulatory factor of BORIS, was bound to CTA's promoter to reciprocally upregulate the level of methylation in lung cancer cells [13]. The balance between CTCF and BORIS activities may be central to CTA expression regulation. A non-specific polycomb repressive complex (PRC) inhibitor, such as 3-Deazaneplanocin A (DZNep), has been shown to disrupt the balance of CTAs expression and subsequently induce T cell-mediated cell lysis of lung cancer cells [10]. Vaccines targeting CTAs induce T cell mediated antitumor immunity has been observed in melanoma [14]. Modulating epigenetic environment through immunogenic target such as CTA provided a new therapeutic approach to cancer therapy.

In addition to gene regulation by modifying the epigenetic microenvironment, hypomethylation can also occur globally, promoting chromosomal instability in cancer cells. This process begins with reactivation of transposable elements that are commonly seen in cancers [15]. Transposable elements typically contain repetitive nucleotides and a high frequency of CpG dinucleotides. Methylation of transposable elements correlates nicely with the degree of global methyhlation status. Using a NF1 mutation mouse model, induced genome-wide hypomethylation is associated with increased chromosomal instability that subsequently lead to a variety of genomic alterations such as deletion or translocation [16].

This relationship was also observed in human cancers where satellite DNA's are frequently hypomethylated near their pericentromeric domain leading to accelerated DNA rearrangements in the regions [17]. Beyond the disturbance at the molecular level, the genome wide hypomethylation is implicated in clinical application. Analysis of 364 samples from patients with NSCLC revealed that the presence of hypomethylated repetitive long interspersed nucleotide element-1(LINE-1) is an independent poor prognostic indicator in early stage NSCLC [18]. Investigation of the methylation mechanism for transposable elements will elucidate our understanding of a phenomenon of genome instability during cancer progression.

DNA Hypermethylation

Although global DNA hypomethylation was the first epigenetic change discovered in cancer, the most extensively studied epigenetic alteration over the last two decades is promoter region hypermethylation [19,20]. Our understanding of hypermethylating alterations began with the study of imprinting genetic disorders, which later connected epigenetic dysregulation to human cancers [21-23]. Beckwith-Wiedemann Syndrome (BWS) is an imprinting growth disorder that is a result of gene hypermethylation dysregulation at a region containing genes, IGF2 and H19[24]. By analyzing a large patient registry with BWS, H19 hypermethylation and loss of imprinting (LOI) of IGF2 were linked to increased risk of BWS defect [25]. Subsequent studies showed that H19 and IGF2 are reciprocally imprinted, leading to paternal expression of IGF2 and maternal of H19 in Wilm's tumor [26-28]. Since its discovery, IGF2 has been associated with many malignancies including lung cancers. However, IGF2 over-expression (or loss of imprinting) by itself is not sufficient to promote tumor transformation [29-31]. An interesting observation in a lung cancer cell line showed that IGF2 might carry out both local and long-range interaction with chromosomal regions [30]. It raises the potential explanation of how IGF2 and H19 imprinting may disrupt gene regulation of multiple pathways leading to tumor transformation. Other LOI of genes in lung cancer includes PEG1/MEST which is seen more frequently in NSCLC than in SCLC cell lines, suggesting that cellular differentiation and histological differences affect epigenetics (similar to the impact of different histologic types on genetic ones) at the molecular level of lung cancer biology [32].

As discussed earlier, DNA methylation is catalyzed by DNMT, an enzyme unique to eukaryotic cells. There are three known DNMTs in mammalian cells: DNMT3a/3b, DNMT2, and DNMT1. DNMT3a and DNMT3b are responsible for de novo DNA methylation while DNMT1 is responsible for maintaining methylation pattern during DNA replication. DNMT2 protein showed relatively low level of activity and has now been shown to mediate tRNA methylation. The study of CpG island methylation has been an area of intense focus in cancer research because of the ability to transcriptionally silence genes. One of the early discoveries of DNA hypermethylation affecting a cancer related gene was made by examining calcitonin silencing in small-cell lung cancers [33]. Since the discovery of the relationship between DNA methylation and transcriptional silencing, hypermethylation has been accepted as a key element in inactivating tumor suppressor genes in cancer development. One example is the Ras associated domain family 1A gene (RASSF1A) [34]. It is located on the short arm of chromosome 3 in a region that frequently undergoes loss of heterozygosity mutation in human malignancy, particularly in SCLC and to a lesser extent in NSCLC. Interestingly extensive search for mutational inactivation of genes located in this region was unproductive. RASSF1A, however, is rarely mutated in cancer, suggesting an alternative explanation for its dysfunction. It turns out that silencing of RASSF1A gene is mediated by promoter hypermethylation. More than 70% of RASSF1A was reported to be hypermethylated in SCLC and about 20-40% in NSCLC [35]. Spontaneous tumorigensis in RASSF1A knockout mouse supports its function as a tumor suppressor gene [36]. P16/INK, a CDK4 inhibitor, is another well studied example of a tumor suppressor gene that demonstrates frequent hypermethylation-mediated gene silencing in lung cancer.

The catalog of genes undergoing tumor-associated DNA hypermethylation continues to grow as our technology advances in screening candidate tumor suppressors. The hypermethylated genes implicated as tumor suppressors are responsible for various essential cellular regulatory pathways including self-sufficient growth signaling, DNA repair mechanism, apoptosis control, cell adhesion/metastasis as well as other critical aspects of cancer development (Table 1) [23,37-40]. O6-methylguanine-DNA-methyl transferase (MGMT) is a frequently hypermethylated and, therefore, silenced gene in lung cancer that functions as a DNA repair gene in normal cells.

Table 1. Hypermethylated genes in lung cancers

Function	Genes
Signal transduction/ Growth factor response	RASSF1A*, CRABP2, IGFBP3*, MAP2K3, TSLC1, RAR beta, BRCA1, BRCA2, EGFR, PTEN, SOCS1, SOCS3, BMP3B, ER, PAX5 a/b*
Apoptosis	DAP-kinase, DcR1, DcR2, ASC/TMS1*
Cell adhesion	T-cadherin*, E-cadherin* , H-cadeherin*
Metastasis	TIMP3*, TIMP4, CXCL12*, APC*, DAPK*
Cell cycle regulation	CDKN2A*(p16/INK4a), CDKN2A (p14/ARF), FHIT*, P15, RB, Caspase 8, CHFR, BLU, 14-3-3sigma
DNA repair	MGMT*, MLH1*, MLH2, GSTP1
Axon guidance	SEMA, SLIT2
Polyamine metabolism	MTAP
Tumor suppressors	SRBC, MYO18B, DLEC1*

*hypermethylated genes that are prognostic in lung cancer.

Ras-association domain family 1 protein, isoform A (RASSF1A), cellular retinoic acid-binding protein 2 (CRABP2), insulin-like growth factor binding protein-3 (IGFBP3), mitogen-activated protein kinase kinase 3 (MAP2K3), tumour suppressor in lung cancer 1 (TSLC1), retinoic acid receptor-beta (RAR beta), breast cancer (BRCA), epidermal growth factor receptor (EGFR), phosphatase and tensin homolog (PTEN), suppressor of cytokine signaling (SOCS), bone morphogenetic protein 3B (BMP3B), estrogen receptor (ER), paired box 5 (PAX5), death-associated protein (DAP), decoy receptor (DcR), apoptosis-associated speck-like protein containing a caspase recruitment domain (ASC), target of methylation-induced silencing 1 (TMS1), tissue inhibitor of metalloproteinases (TIMP), C-X-C chemokine ligand 12 (CXCL12), adenomatous polyposis coli (APC), death-associated protein kinase (DAPK), cyclin-dependent kinase (CDK), fragile histidine triad (FHIT), retinoblastoma (Rb), checkpoint gene with forkhead-associated domain and ring finger (CHFR), a candidate tumor suppressor gene (BLU), O(6)-methylguanine DNA methyltransferase (MGMT), mutL homolog (MLH), glutathione s-transferase P1 (GSTP1), semaphorin (SEMA), a candidate tumor suppressor gene (SLIT), methylthioadenosine phosphorylase (MTAP), serum deprivation response factor (sdr)-related gene product (SRBC), candidate tumor suppresors of myosin family (MYO18B), deleted in lung and esophageal cancer 1 (DLEC1).

Hypermethylation of hMLH1 gene (involved in DNA repair) and CDKN2A or TP53 (involved in cell cycle regulation) have been observed in many solid tumors including lung cancers. Aberrant methylation of E-Cadherin and H-Cadherin genes that modulate the epithelial to mesenchymal phenotype is associated with higher risk of tumor invasion in NSCLC[38,39,41,42]. Epithelial cell differentiation is kept in check by surrounding environment such as intercellular adhesions. The number of putative tumor suppressor genes that are inactivated by epigenetic modification may actually be more than those inactivated through genetic mutations[43]. This statement forces a new perspective in our orientation of human genetics and highlights the global effects of epigenetic modification in cancer biology.

Histone Modification

Histone modifications help maintain a complex and dynamic chromatin environment. This can be explained by a simplified model of two functional states of chromatin structures: euchromatin where areas of DNA is made accessible to transcription, or heterochromatin where DNA is inaccessible. The balance of these two states is key during DNA replication and condensation. Similar processes also occur more locally during gene transcription and repair. In order to carry out these reactions, a cascade of events to assemble the necessary machinery must happen.

As discussed earlier, hypermethylation is associated with transcriptional silencing of genes. The cascade of transcriptional silencing appears to start with methylation of CpG islands in a promoter region which subsequently recruits methyl DNA binding proteins such as methyl-CpG binding protein 2 (MeCP2) and methyl binding domain protein 2 (MBD2), as well as histone deacetylase (HDACs). This multiprotein complex renders promoter regions inaccessible to transcriptional proteins, thereby resulting in transcription repression. Among the assembly of proteins, HDAC, in particular, recognizes the acetyl group attached to the lysine residues in the tails of a histone molecule. This post translational modification of the N terminal tail of histone (removal of the acetyl group usually followed by histone methylation), promotes DNA condensation and a repressive structure [44]. Deacetylation by HDACs, like many other balanced biological systems is countered by an opposing reaction of histone acetyl transferase (HAT) enzymes which add acetyl groups to the histones tail permitting recruitment of chromatin remodeling factors and gene transcription. DNA de-methyation, together with post translational modification such as histone de-acetylation oversees in chromatin regulations that either inhibit or enable transcriptional activity [45].

The mechanism that involves in the switching between the two transcriptional states has only recently begun to be understood. Polycomb group proteins (PCG) are essential epigenetic regulators for stem cell growth and renewal [46]. There are two major types of polycomb repressive complexes, PRC1 and PRC2, which function in conjunction with each other to repress gene transcription. PRC2 protein complexes contain a catalytic component, EZH2, which can directly interact with DNMTs. There is evidence that EZH2 is able to recruit methylation protein complex and facilitate gene suppression[47]. PRC1, on the other hand, contains a BMI-1 catalytic subunit that is important in maintaining gene silencing through its ability to read repressive histone markers, such as H3K9me3 and H3K27me3 [48].

EZH2 and BMI1 together are over expressed in various types of tumors, including lung cancers, and are often associated with poor prognosis [49].

While DNA methylation and histone modification are critical processes in gene regulation, there is a more global epigenetic influence, modulated by chromatin remodeling complex, at work. Enzymatic activity of chromatin remodeling complex can mobilize nucleosomes by inserting or removing histone octamers. Through nucleosome repositioning, the complex can control accessibility of DNA binding factors and interact with other chromatin structures. One such class of family is SWI/SNF complex that has been associated with numerous tumor suppressor genes in human cancers [50]. BRG1/BRM are ATPase subunits of SWI/SNF protein complex. The loss of BRG1 and BRM expression was seen in 30% of NSCLC and has been implicated in lung cancer tumorogenesis [51,52].

Epigenetic and Lung Cancer Stem Cell

The concept of cancer stem cells (CSC) originates from the observation that tumors consist of heterogeneous populations with various function and morphology. The cell populations have diverse tumorigenic capacities with cancer stem cells at the top of the hierarchy [53]. This subgroup of cancer cells is able to generate differentiated tumor cells and are resistant to cytotoxic agents. The CSCs retain their stem-cell like abilities that may be responsible for cancer recurrence, resistance and metastasis [54].

The first study that bought up the cancer stem cell hypothesis originated from examining patients with acute myeloid leukemia. The study demonstrated that leukemic cells possessing phenotypic features of hematopoietic stem cells[55]. Growing evidence in animal models and observation of solid cancer behavior supports the relevance of cancer stem cell hypothesis.

The interest in lung cancer stem cells research was piqued by the ability of pluripotent pulmonary epithelial cells to maintain their stem-cells like features[56]. Gene silencing is mediated by epigenetic modulation via mechanism such as DNA methylation, chromatin modification and histone remodeling. When epithelial cells are under environmental stress which can disturb the homeostasis of epigenetic environment, gene transcription can be turned on or off during cell renewal and proliferation. Prolonged exposure to environmental stimulus, such as chronic inflammation common in a smoker, can lead to abnormal expansion which favors clonal cells that can proliferate rather than differentiate[57]. This survival advantage allows accumulations of additional epigenetic and genetic changes that eventually lead to tumor transformation. Our understanding of CSC in lung cancer came from the study of Clara cells regeneration in a lung injury mouse model. The exposure to naphthalene leads to the ablation of Clara cells which triggers bronchoalveolar stem cells (BASCs) self renewal. BASCs have been recognized as a critical player of tumorigenesis in adenocarcinoma[57]. Studies examining KRAS mutations, p38 or PTEN knockout mouse model all had similar observations of increased proliferation of BASCs in animals carrying these mutations. The transformed BASCs are more prone to expand and proliferate after external stimulus such as that seen in injured lung epithelium. Polycomb proteins (discussed earlier) are fundamental epigenetic regulators in maintaining the characteristics of stem cells[58]. Ablating the function of EZH2 and BMI1 can deprive cancer cells' ability to maintain stem cell properties and prevent tumor formation. In lung cancer cell lines, non-specific PRC inhibitor has shown pre-clinical efficacy in reversing polycomb-mediated gene silencing[10]. More specific agents may be available in the future that can reintroduce normal suppression of embryonic genes in cancer stem cells. Pharmacologic targeting of PRCs may be an emerging novel strategy in cancer therapy.

Epigenetic and Airway Diseases

Recent examination of prenatal tobacco exposure and neonatal buccal cell DNA methylation pattern highlights the importance of environmental exposure and methylation modulation[59] (Figure 1). Indeed, chronic inflammation associated with smoking has long been associated with the development of chronic obstructive pulmonary disorder (COPD) and carcinogenesis [60]. The understanding of epigenetic processes has shed a distinct light on the complex mechanisms behind chronic inflammation and cellular transformation at the molecular level[61].

Increased oxidant release from activated macrophages, neutrophils and lymphocytes can be triggered by carcinogenic exposure as seen in smokers [62]. The exposed tissues, through regulation of transcription factor nuclear factor kappa B (NK-kB), release pro-inflammatory signals such as IL-6, IL-8 and TNF-alpha [63,64]. NK-kB is a critical player in inducing inflammatory gene expression. It has the ability to recruit co-activator and histone remodeling complex such as HDACs and HATs. Subtle fluctuation in the temporal profile of NK-kB activation can have profound effects on its surrounding epigenetic environment [65]. COPD patients can have significantly depressed HDAC activity level that correlates with the severity of the disease [61,66].

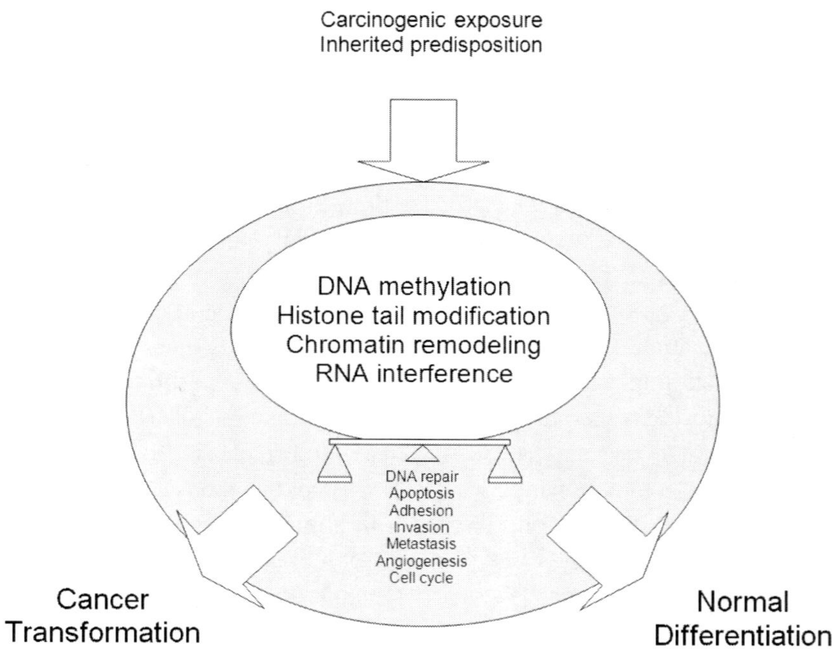

Figure 1. Environmental exposure and epigenetic changes.

It has been postulated that, glucocorticoids and theophylline (which is a HDAC activator) may exerts its anti-inflammatory effect by restoring HDAC activity in COPD patients [66].

The renewal and proliferation of pulmonary epithelial cells relies upon an overlapping network of regulatory pathways that include Wnt, Hedghog and Notch signaling pathways [42]. The Wnt pathway, regulated by an inhibitory protein, secreted frizzled-related protein (SFRP), has been studied extensively in colorectal cancer. SFRP is epigenetically silenced in normal epithelium. When this suppression is lifted, Beta-catenin transcription, downstream of Wnt signaling, activates MYC and cyclin D that in turn promotes cell proliferation and survival [67]. Although tumor development in lung cancer was not thought to be a lineage step-wise progression, similar activation of the Wnt pathway has been observed in NSCLC. Manipulation of the transcription factor GATA, a Wnt signaling antagonist, ablated Wnt signaling has been found to promote BASC transformation [68,69].

Noncoding RNAs

First described in C. elegans, noncoding RNAs have been found to be critical regulators in numerous important biological pathways including cell proliferation, differentiation, and apoptosis. During the short time since their discovery, over 800 miRNAs have been identified; although, its capacity in regulating cancer biology is still under intensive investigation. miRNA regulates its target gene by binding to its partially complementary sequences in the 3' or 5 –untranslated region of the target mRNAs. mRNA and miRNA complex can accelerate the degradation of target mRNA and, therefore, gene suppression post-transcriptionally, as well as translational repression without necessarily causing RNA degradation. Once discovered, investigators quickly found that miRNAs are dysregulated in cancers with both over-expression and under-expression when compared with normal counterparts. miRNAs can therefore function as oncogenic miRNAs (when over-expressed) and tumor suppressive miRNAs (presumably when under-expressed). One of the miRNAs found to be dysregulated in lung cancer is the let-7 product [70]. The RAS oncogene contains multiple complementary sequences in the 3'UTR that serves as a target for let-7 [70]. Reduced function in RAS family has been observed in let-7 expressing tumors. Ectopic expression of RAS can then rescue let-7 mediated tumor suppression. miRNA-128b is another example of microRNA implicated in lung cancer tumorigenesis. It is located on chromosome 3p which is frequently lost as an early genetic event in lung cancer development. Loss of miRNA-128b is linked to increased epidermal growth factor receptor (EGFR) expression (one of the putative targets) and is correlated with treatment response to EGFR tyrosine kinase inhibitors [71]. microRNA can also exert its regulatory function through other epigenetic targets. The miR-29 family has been linked to modulating CpG island methylation pattern in lung cancer cells through targets such as DNMT3A and DNMT3B [72,73]. As the understanding of the regulatory potential of microRNAs grows, it is not surprising to find that miRNA encodes targets in many fundamental cellular pathways. Known miRNAs implicated in lung cancer are listed in Table 2 [74-80]. miRNA frequently has mismatched sequence against its target mRNA. Imperfect matching allows a single miRNA to regulate translation of multiple different genes. In fact, perfect match of a single miRNA may not be sufficient to exert the degree of inhibition observed by the collaboration of multiple miRNAs. With the recent development of high throughput analyses of miRNA expression, several studies have suggested that miRNA expression profile exhibited certain patterns among lung cancers. The expression profile has provided translational researchers new techniques to predict cancer behavior and efficacy of existing therapy. miRNA has also been evaluated for potential therapeutic target. Inhibition of miRNA activity such as administration of anti-miRNA oligonucleotides(AMO) is being explored as novel approach to regulate miRNA function [81]. Conversely, reintroducing miRNA that is known to be suppressed in cancer cells could have therapeutic effects in reversing tumor growth as demonstrated by intranasal administration of let-7 in a lung cancer mouse model [82].

Biomarkers

Various biomarkers are being developed to help cancer diagnosis, to determine prognosis and to assess responsiveness to therapy. Let-7 family is closely associated with early lung cancer development. Decreased let-7 level carries poor prognosis independent of clinical staging of lung cancer [83].

Table 2. miRNA dysregulated in lung cancer

Function	miRNA	Proposed regulatory targets
Apoptosis	↓ miR-1*	MET, Pim-1, FOXP1, HDAC4
	↑ miR-21*	PTEN, PDCD4, Maspin, TPM1
	↓ miR-29	DNMT3A/3B
	↑ miR-221/miR-222	PTEN, TIMP3, c-Kit, p27(kip1)
	↑ let-7*	KRAS, MYC, CDK6, CDC25A, cyclin D2, Lin-28,
Adhesion	↓ miR-200	Flt1/VEGFR1
	↓ miR-126	SLC7A5, VEGF
Proliferation	↑ miR-197/miR-93	FUS1/TUSC2
	↓ miR-31	LATS2, PPP2R2A
	↑ miR-155*	FOXO3A
P53 pathway	↓ miR-34a*	CDK4/6, CCNE2, Axl
	↑ miR-128-2	E2F5
Rb pathway	↑ miR-17-29 cluster	PTEN, CTGF, TSP1, TGFb, E2F, CDKN1A, HIF1a
	↓ miR-15a/miR-16	CCND1, CCND3, CCNE1
EGFR pathway	↓ miR-7	EGFR, Raf1, Akt, ERK
	↑ miR-21	EGFR-activating mutations

*miRNAs that are prognostic in lung cancer ; ↑ oncogenic; ↓ antitumorigenic;

A member of the Provirus integrating site Moloney murine leukemia virus family involves in regulation of cell apoptosis (Pim-1), forkhead box protein (Fox), programmed cell death 4 (PDCD4), a member of the serpin family (Maspin), a thymidylate kinase (TMP1), a putative tumor suppressor belongs to CDKI family (p27(kip1)), cell division cycle 25 homolog A (CDC25A), vascular endothelial growth factor receptors (Flt1/VEGFR1), component of 4F2 amino acid transporter (SLC7A5), vascular endothelial growth factor (VEGF), tumor suppressor candidate 2 (FUS1/TUSC2), large tumor suppressor 2 (LATS2), phosphatase 2A subunit B (PPP2R2A), cyclin (CCN), a receptor tyrosine kinase belongs to the Tyro3, Axl, and Mer family (Axl), cell cycle-related transcription factor 5 (E2F5), connective tissue growth factor (CTGF), thrombospondin-1 (TSP1), transforming growth factor beta (TGFb), hypoxia-inducible factor 1A (HIF1A), a serine-threonine kinase invlves in signal transduction pathways of cell proliferation (Raf1), protein kinase B (Akt), extracellular signal-regulated kinase (ERK).

Expression profile of miRNA from peripheral blood is able to distinguish non-small cell lung cancer from non cancerous samples suggesting clinical utility of circulating miRNA signatures for lung cancer screening [84,85]. Similarly, investigators have suggested that the expression of miR-205 helps to distinguish squamous cancers from non-squamous lung cancers [86]. The miRNA signature is one of many epigenetic diagnostic indicators that is currently under investigation to assist early lung cancer detection. Increasing evidence supports cigarette smoking as a direct contributor to abnormal epigenetic regulation in respiratory epithelial cells and pulmonary carcinogenesis [87]. Persistant epigenetic changes despite smoking cessation suggests the clinical relevance in lung cancer screening strategy [88]. In early studies of p16 and RASSF1A genes, methylation was detected in sputum amongst a high risk population predating the clinical diagnosis of squamous cell carcinoma by 3 years [89]. Mapping the methylation pattern of genes can differentiate high risk lung cancers. Prospective study of 190 chronic smokers revealed that concomitant methylation of a panel of three to six genes predicts 6.5-fold increased risk in future development of lung cancer [90]. Predicting cancer behavior in early stage NSCLC is of particular interest as even with early detection and definitive treatment recurrent disease are seen in more than one third of patients. Risk stratification at the beginning of therapy can potentially direct clinical management among this subset of patients.

A retrospective analysis of early stage NSCLC showed that hypermethylation of four genes, p16, CDH13, APC and RASSF1A in primary tumor and lymph nodes is associated with high risk of recurrence[39]. Promoter methylation of these genes was also detected in regional and mediastinal lymph nodes, suggesting the presence of micrometastases beyond traditional staging by pathologic examination in early stage local disease. This additional molecular information may help guide treatment favoring systemic therapy in early diseases that are associated high risk features. In addition to providing prognostic information, methylation status has been shown to predict response to chemotherapy. The detection of a frequently methylated DNA repair gene, MGMT, in glioma predicts survival and response to treatments with akylating agent [91]. Similar clinical utilization of biomarker in lung cancer has been examined in a retrospective study of aberrant methylation of a G2-M checkpoint control gene, 14-3-3sigma. Silencing of 14-3-3sigma by hypermethylation is associated with improved disease control in cisplatin/gemcitabine treated advanced NSCLC[92].

Expression profile of miRNA has also been extensively studied in predicting response to treatment among lung cancer patients. A panel consisting of 5 miRNAs - two exhibiting protective effects (miR-221, let-7) and three indicative of high risk disease (miR-137, miR-372, miR-182), demonostrated strong prognostic value for treatment outcome and survival in NSCLC[93].

Epigenetic Therapeutics

DNMT Inhibitors

Epigenetic changes are fundamentally different from genetic mutations in that they are reversible events. Strategies to exploit these reversible epigenetic changes in cancer cells represent an attractive approach in cancer therapy. Tumorigenesis typically occurs through the accumulation of genetic and epigenetic neoplastic-prone features such as impaired DNA repair mechanism, the loss of signals in apoptosis, or gaining the ability of sustaining signals to multiply. Since epigenetic modulation has such broad effects in cellular physiology, our ability to reverse the machinery can have profound effects on the process of tumorigenesis. One such example is the discovery that certain cytosine analogues, 5-azacytidine and 5-aza-2'-deoxycytidine (decitabine) functioned not merely as antimetabolites, but that they were effective DNA methyltransferase inhibitor. These agents are cytidine and deoxycytidine analogs respectively that are incorporated into DNA sequence during DNA replication. During the enzymatic reaction of methyl group transfer, base containing 5-azacytidine and 5-aza-2'-deoxycytidine binds to DNMTs covalently thereby rendering DNMT inactive. Because of their dependence on DNA replication, DNMT inhibitors are S-phase-specific agents. In preclinical settings, decitabine has been shown to re-express silenced gene by decreasing methylation in cancer cell lines [94,95]. Similar results were confirmed in multiple lung cancer mouse models [96]. Demethylating agents were first used in clinical setting in hematologic malignancies [97]. Toxicity such as myelosuppresion was a common problem amongst patients treated with these agents in early studies and remained a problem until relatively low dose regimens were developed [98,99]. Investigators subsequently showed that low dose chronic exposure seemed to produce improved results consistent with the underlying biology suggesting that prolonging the S-phase exposure should produce better outcome. Momparler et al showed 1 out of 9 patients with metastatic lung cancers had prolonged survival (81 months) in a dose-finding phase I trials for decitabine (8 h intravenous infusion of 200–660 mg/m2). They found a median survival of 6.7 months, with three patients surviving more than 15 months [100]. One recent trial using low dose decitabine observed no clinical response in 32 patients with lung cancers [101].

The resistance observed in platinum-based therapy follows a dose-response curve with flattening at higher dose. It is postulated that the resistance can be introduced by hypermethylation-mediated gene silencing of DNA repair genes or drug transporter such as CTR21 [102]. Schwartsmann et al examined the combination of decitabine (67 mg/m2) with cisplatin (33mg/m2) in patients with inoperable NSCLC. Three minor responses were observed among 9 patients enrolled in the study with a median survivals of 15 weeks [103]. In many of the studies, attempts were made to measure the effects of demethylation through surrogate markers such as fetal hemoglobin expression and MAGE1A CpG island in buccal cells. Methylation was decreased with exposure to demethylating agents even after one cycle of treatment [104]. Shrump et al obtained serial FNAs of the tumor mass following each cycle of decitabine to assess treatment response within the tumor's microenvironment [101]. Microarray data of these samples showed corresponding up regulation of CTAs after decitabine treatment. This finding may provide an interesting rationale for immunotherapy exploiting immunogenic CTAs in lung cancer patients in a combination therapy with demethylating agents.

HDAC Inhibitors

At least 18 HDACs have been identified with various functions [44,105]. They are subdivided into four classes based on their activities and cellular compartment. Class I HDACs are expressed in the nucleus and are ubiquitous in all cell types. Class II HDACs can shuttle between nucleus and the cytoplasm while Class IIb HDACs are expressed only in cytoplasm and function specifically in regulating cytoskeletal proteins. The class III HDACs are homologous to the yeast Sir2 protein which is responsible for cellular response to redox status. Class IV HDACs shared similar enzymatic activities as class I and II which are functionally dependent on zinc molecules at the active binding site.

Histone modifications are just as critical as DNA methylation in regulating gene expression. Deacetylation at the lysine tail of histone promotes a condensed chromatin configuration that renders DNA sequence inaccessible for transcriptional machinery. HDAC inhibition can lead to unwinding of the chromatin and reactivate previously silenced genes. Hypoacetylated histones are common findings in cancer cell lines [106]. Therefore, there has been considerable effort to develop agents that target HDACs and theoretically reverse aberrant epigenetic changes [107].

Interestingly, HDAC inhibitors might have far more extensive biological roles than had been anticipated. Various non-histone proteins have been identified as HDAC substrates including p53, p73, C-MYC, RUNX3, HIF-1a, and HSP90 to name a few [108]. HDAC inhibitors (perhaps a more appropriate term would be protein deacetylase inhibitors), through their pervasive influence on cellular regulatory pathways (nucleosomal as well as non-nucleosomal), are able to control cell differentiation, apoptosis, DNA repair and replications.

There are several HDAC inhibitors that are in clinical development, including vorinostat, etinostat, romidepsin, valproic acid, hydralazine, phenylbutyrate, LBH589, and CUDC-101 [109]. Vorinostat is an FDA approved oral agent as a third-line monotherapy for cutaneous T-cell lymphoma[110]. A phase II study of 14 patients examined the effects of single agent vorinostat in advanced NSCLC [111]. No objective antitumor responses were observed but 8 patients experienced stable disease. The study suggested that the low rate of antitumor response was likely due to vorinostat's characteristic as a biologic response modifier rather than a cytotoxic drug. The author hypothesized that the most benefit would be derived with combination of HDAC inhibitor with other anticancer agents. A phase I trial examined the combination of Vorinostat with carboplatin and paclitaxel in patients with advanced solid tumors [112]. Ten of 19 patients with advanced NSCLC experienced partial response and additional four had stable disease (overall 73%). A follow up phase II placebo-controlled study examined this combination in ninety-four patients who were randomized to carboplatin plus pactlitaxel with either Vorinostat (400mg by mouth daily) or placebo. Response rate was 34% among patients who received vorinostat compared to 12.5% in the placebo arm. There is a trend toward improved PFS (6.0 months versus 4.1 months) and OS (13.0 months versus 9.7 months) [113]. Its subsequent phase III randomized trial of 253 patients, however, was closed early for futility in the vorinostat arm [114].

Romidepsin is another potent inhibitor of HDAC that has a bicyclic peptide structure. Nineteen patients with refractory lung cancer (16 NSCLC's and 3 SCLC's) were treated with romidepsin 17.8mg/m2 infusions on day 1 and 8 of a 21 day cycle. There was transient stabilization of disease in nine patients but no objective responses were observed [115]. A phase II trial examining romidepsin as a single agent in relapsed SCLC's was similarly disappointing [116]. Despite no clinical response when used as monotherapy, there was interesting preclinical data demonstrating enhanced effect when combined with erlotinib [116-118]. Romidepsin can sensitize NSCLC cell lines to erolotinb but also restore EGFR-TKI sensitivity after developing resistance suggesting again that combinatory therapy may help us derive the most benefit from epigenetic therapy [119].

While single agent activity of epigenetic modulating agents in solid tumor has in general been disappointing, we have observed interesting synergism by inhibiting both the enzymatic activities of methylation and deacetylation in vitro and in vivo [120,121]. This strategy of disrupting cancerous epigenetic environment at various targets simultaneously has been examined in recent clinical trials. A phase II study of 17 patients with refractory solid tumors examined the combination of hydralazine (an oral antihypertensive also a weak DMNT inhibitor) and decitabine while receiving standard chemotherapy treatment. Twelve of 15 patients (80%) had clinical benefits. Valproic acid is a commonly used anticonvulsant that is also a modestly potent HDAC inhibitors at therapeutic blood concentration [122]. It produces disease control when combining with doxorubicin in treating refractory malignant mesothelioma [123]. A phase I study of valproic acid in combination with decitabine in advanced NSCLC did not show clinical response and was closed early due to grade 3 or 4 neurological toxicity [124]. Clinical trials examined various combinations of DNMT and HDAC inihibitors; for example, hydralazine and magnesium valproate, 5-azacytidine and valproic acid, and sodium phenylbutyrate and 5-azacytidine combinations. Although these trials were based on plausible hypothesis, synergism of HDAC and DNMT inhibition has not been observed in the clinical setting [125-128].

Conclusion

Our understanding of tumor biology has changed significantly over the past 30 years. Genetic mutations and epigenetic alterations together govern a complex interaction of DNA and chromatin modification. Gene expression or suppression modulated by this network provides lung cancer with phenotypic features such as histology, prognosis and responsiveness to therapy. Environmental stimulus and cellular stressors can shift the epigenetic machinery favoring cancer development and acquiring stem cell-like features; however, the exact mechanism and its downstream effectors remain to be elucidated. Knowing the functional components of epigenetic changes will provide potential molecular targets for therapy. In addition to finding new therapeutic targets, examining existing therapy utilizing DNMT or HDAC inhibitors and fine tuning various combination therapy or developing narrower targeted inhibitors are of great interest. With recent development of high–throughput technologies and mapping of cancer epigenome [129], we are able to identify variations of epigenetic components that will allow development of molecular markers for early detection, prediction of prognosis and response to treatment in our approach toward personalized medicine.

From the recognition of CpG islands alteration in the early 80's to unraveling the multiple layers of epigenetic dysregulation, we have come a long way in a quest to decipher the significance of epigenetics in lung cancer biology. The field of epigenetics is maturing and our view of cancer biology can no longer consider genetic alterations as a separate entity from epigenetic. As we move forward in translating our knowledge to clinical practice, only by reminding ourselves of the intercalated network of epigenetic and genetic, can we succeed in our fight against lung cancer.

References

[1] 1999–2007 Cancer Incidence and Mortality Data, in Department of Health and Human Services CfDCaP, and National Cancer Institute (ed). Atlanta, U.S. Cancer Statistics Working Group, 2010.

[2] Jones PA, Baylin SB: The fundamental role of epigenetic events in cancer. *Nat. Rev. Genet.* 3:415-28, 2002.

[3] Baylin SB, Jones PA: A decade of exploring the cancer epigenome - biological and translational implications. *Nat. Rev. Cancer.* 11:726-34, 2011.

[4] Futscher BW, Oshiro MM, Wozniak RJ, et al: Role for DNA methylation in the control of cell type specific maspin expression. *Nat. Genet.* 31:175-9, 2002.

[5] Fraga MF, Ballestar E, Villar-Garea A, et al: Loss of acetylation at Lys16 and trimethylation at Lys20 of histone H4 is a common hallmark of human cancer. *Nat. Genet.* 37:391-400, 2005.

[6] Takai D, Jones PA: Comprehensive analysis of CpG islands in human chromosomes 21 and 22. *Proc. Natl. Acad. Sci. U S A.* 99:3740-5, 2002.

[7] Feinberg AP, Vogelstein B: Hypomethylation distinguishes genes of some human cancers from their normal counterparts. *Nature.* 301:89-92, 1983.

[8] Goelz SE, Vogelstein B, Hamilton SR, et al: Hypomethylation of DNA from benign and malignant human colon neoplasms. *Science.* 228:187-90, 1985.

[9] Gure AO, Chua R, Williamson B, et al: Cancer-testis genes are coordinately expressed and are markers of poor outcome in non-small cell lung cancer. *Clin. Cancer Res.* 11:8055-62, 2005.

[10] Rao M, Chinnasamy N, Hong JA, et al: Inhibition of histone lysine methylation enhances cancer-testis antigen expression in lung cancer cells: implications for adoptive immunotherapy of cancer. *Cancer Res.* 71:4192-204, 2011.

[11] Glazer CA, Smith IM, Ochs MF, et al: Integrative discovery of epigenetically derepressed cancer testis antigens in NSCLC. *PLoS One.* 4:e8189, 2009.

[12] Bhan S, Negi SS, Shao C, et al: BORIS binding to the promoters of cancer testis antigens, MAGEA2, MAGEA3, and MAGEA4, is associated with their transcriptional activation in lung cancer. *Clin. Cancer Res.* 17:4267-76, 2011.

[13] Hong JA, Kang Y, Abdullaev Z, et al: Reciprocal binding of CTCF and BORIS to the NY-ESO-1 promoter coincides with derepression of this cancer-testis gene in lung cancer cells. *Cancer Res.* 65:7763-74, 2005.

[14] Sigalotti L, Fratta E, Coral S, et al: Intratumor heterogeneity of cancer/testis antigens expression in human cutaneous melanoma is methylation-regulated and functionally reverted by 5-aza-2'-deoxycytidine. *Cancer Res.* 64:9167-71, 2004.

[15] Wilson AS, Power BE, Molloy PL: DNA hypomethylation and human diseases. *Biochim. Biophys. Acta.* 1775:138-62, 2007.

[16] Eden A, Gaudet F, Waghmare A, et al: Chromosomal instability and tumors promoted by DNA hypomethylation. *Science.* 300:455, 2003.

[17] Wong N, Lam WC, Lai PB, et al: Hypomethylation of chromosome 1 heterochromatin DNA correlates with q-arm copy gain in human hepatocellular carcinoma. *Am. J. Pathol.* 159:465-71, 2001.

[18] Saito K, Kawakami K, Matsumoto I, et al: Long interspersed nuclear element 1 hypomethylation is a marker of poor prognosis in stage IA non-small cell lung cancer. *Clin. Cancer Res.* 16:2418-26, 2010.
[19] Herman JG, Baylin SB: Gene silencing in cancer in association with promoter hypermethylation. *N. Engl. J. Med.* 349:2042-54, 2003.
[20] Feinberg AP, Tycko B: The history of cancer epigenetics. *Nat. Rev. Cancer.* 4:143-53, 2004.
[21] Kondo M, Takahashi T: [Altered genomic imprinting in the IGF2 and H19 genes in human lung cancer]. *Nihon. Rinsho.* 54:492-6, 1996.
[22] Rainier S, Johnson LA, Dobry CJ, et al: Relaxation of imprinted genes in human cancer. *Nature.* 362:747-9, 1993.
[23] Suzuki H, Ueda R, Takahashi T: Altered imprinting in lung cancer. *Nat. Genet.* 6:332-3, 1994.
[24] Engel JR, Smallwood A, Harper A, et al: Epigenotype-phenotype correlations in Beckwith-Wiedemann syndrome. *J. Med. Genet.* 37:921-6, 2000.
[25] DeBaun MR, Niemitz EL, McNeil DE, et al: Epigenetic alterations of H19 and LIT1 distinguish patients with Beckwith-Wiedemann syndrome with cancer and birth defects. *Am. J. Hum. Genet.* 70:604-11, 2002.
[26] Moulton T, Crenshaw T, Hao Y, et al: Epigenetic lesions at the H19 locus in Wilms' tumour patients. *Nat. Genet.* 7:440-7, 1994.
[27] Steenman MJ, Rainier S, Dobry CJ, et al: Loss of imprinting of IGF2 is linked to reduced expression and abnormal methylation of H19 in Wilms' tumour. *Nat. Genet.* 7:433-9, 1994.
[28] Li L, Keverne EB, Aparicio SA, et al: Regulation of maternal behavior and offspring growth by paternally expressed Peg3. *Science.* 284:330-3, 1999.
[29] Holm TM, Jackson-Grusby L, Brambrink T, et al: Global loss of imprinting leads to widespread tumorigenesis in adult mice. *Cancer Cell.* 8:275-85, 2005.
[30] Vu TH, Nguyen AH, Hoffman AR: Loss of IGF2 imprinting is associated with abrogation of long-range intrachromosomal interactions in human cancer cells. *Hum. Mol. Genet.* 19:901-19, 2010.
[31] Rogler CE, Yang D, Rossetti L, et al: Altered body composition and increased frequency of diverse malignancies in insulin-like growth factor-II transgenic mice. *J. Biol. Chem.* 269:13779-84, 1994.
[32] Nakanishi H, Suda T, Katoh M, et al: Loss of imprinting of PEG1/MEST in lung cancer cell lines. Oncol Rep 12:1273-8, 2004.
[33] Baylin SB, Hoppener JW, de Bustros A, et al: DNA methylation patterns of the calcitonin gene in human lung cancers and lymphomas. *Cancer Res.* 46:2917-22, 1986.
[34] Pfeifer GP, Dammann R: Methylation of the tumor suppressor gene RASSF1A in human tumors. *Biochemistry.* (Mosc) 70:576-83, 2005.
[35] Pfeifer GP, Rauch TA: DNA methylation patterns in lung carcinomas. *Semin. Cancer Biol.* 19:181-7, 2009.
[36] Tommasi S, Dammann R, Zhang Z, et al: Tumor susceptibility of Rassf1a knockout mice. *Cancer Res.* 65:92-8, 2005.
[37] Tsou JA, Hagen JA, Carpenter CL, et al: DNA methylation analysis: a powerful new tool for lung cancer diagnosis. *Oncogene.* 21:5450-61, 2002.

[38] Schrump DS, Nguyen DM: Targeting the epigenome for the treatment and prevention of lung cancer. *Semin. Oncol.* 32:488-502, 2005.

[39] Brock MV, Hooker CM, Ota-Machida E, et al: DNA methylation markers and early recurrence in stage I lung cancer. *N Engl. J. Med.* 358:1118-28, 2008.

[40] Gu J, Berman D, Lu C, et al: Aberrant promoter methylation profile and association with survival in patients with non-small cell lung cancer. *Clin. Cancer Res.* 12:7329-38, 2006.

[41] Suzuki M, Yoshino I: Aberrant methylation in non-small cell lung cancer. *Surg. Today.* 40:602-7, 2010.

[42] Sato M, Shames DS, Gazdar AF, et al: A translational view of the molecular pathogenesis of lung cancer. *J. Thorac. Oncol.* 2:327-43, 2007.

[43] Baylin SB, Ohm JE: Epigenetic gene silencing in cancer - a mechanism for early oncogenic pathway addiction? *Nat. Rev. Cancer.* 6:107-16, 2006.

[44] Lane AA, Chabner BA: Histone deacetylase inhibitors in cancer therapy. *J. Clin. Oncol.* 27:5459-68, 2009.

[45] Kouzarides T: Chromatin modifications and their function. *Cell.* 128:693-705, 2007.

[46] Crea F, Paolicchi E, Marquez VE, et al: Polycomb genes and cancer: Time for clinical application? *Crit. Rev. Oncol. Hematol.*, 2011.

[47] Croonquist PA, Van Ness B: The polycomb group protein enhancer of zeste homolog 2 (EZH 2) is an oncogene that influences myeloma cell growth and the mutant ras phenotype. *Oncogene.* 24:6269-80, 2005.

[48] Mohammad HP, Cai Y, McGarvey KM, et al: Polycomb CBX7 promotes initiation of heritable repression of genes frequently silenced with cancer-specific DNA hypermethylation. *Cancer Res.* 69:6322-30, 2009.

[49] Yoon KA, Gil HJ, Han J, et al: Genetic polymorphisms in the polycomb group gene EZH2 and the risk of lung cancer. *J. Thorac. Oncol.* 5:10-6, 2010.

[50] Wilson BG, Roberts CW: SWI/SNF nucleosome remodellers and cancer. *Nat. Rev. Cancer.* 11:481-92, 2011.

[51] Girard L, Zochbauer-Muller S, Virmani AK, et al: Genome-wide allelotyping of lung cancer identifies new regions of allelic loss, differences between small cell lung cancer and non-small cell lung cancer, and loci clustering. *Cancer Res.* 60:4894-906, 2000.

[52] Reisman DN, Sciarrotta J, Wang W, et al: Loss of BRG1/BRM in human lung cancer cell lines and primary lung cancers: correlation with poor prognosis. *Cancer Res.* 63:560-6, 2003.

[53] Tsai HC, Baylin SB: Cancer epigenetics: linking basic biology to clinical medicine. *Cell Res.* 21:502-17, 2011.

[54] Eramo A, Haas TL, De Maria R: Lung cancer stem cells: tools and targets to fight lung cancer. *Oncogene.* 29:4625-35, 2010.

[55] Lapidot T, Sirard C, Vormoor J, et al: A cell initiating human acute myeloid leukaemia after transplantation into SCID mice. *Nature.* 367:645-8, 1994.

[56] Widschwendter M, Fiegl H, Egle D, et al: Epigenetic stem cell signature in cancer. *Nat. Genet.* 39:157-8, 2007.

[57] Gomperts BN, Spira A, Massion PP, et al: Evolving concepts in lung carcinogenesis. *Semin. Respir. Crit. Care Med.* 32:32-43, 2011.

[58] Valk-Lingbeek ME, Bruggeman SW, van Lohuizen M: Stem cells and cancer; the polycomb connection. *Cell.* 118:409-18, 2004.

[59] Breton CV, Byun HM, Wenten M, et al: Prenatal tobacco smoke exposure affects global and gene-specific DNA methylation. *Am. J. Respir. Crit. Care Med.* 180:462-7, 2009.

[60] Adcock IM, Ford P, Ito K, et al: Epigenetics and airways disease. *Respir. Res.* 7:21, 2006.

[61] Ito K, Ito M, Elliott WM, et al: Decreased histone deacetylase activity in chronic obstructive pulmonary disease. *N. Engl. J. Med.* 352:1967-76, 2005.

[62] Herceg Z, Vaissiere T: Epigenetic mechanisms and cancer: an interface between the environment and the genome. *Epigenetics.* 6:804-19, 2011.

[63] Rahman I: Oxidative stress, chromatin remodeling and gene transcription in inflammation and chronic lung diseases. *J. Biochem. Mol. Biol.* 36:95-109, 2003.

[64] Yang SR, Chida AS, Bauter MR, et al: Cigarette smoke induces proinflammatory cytokine release by activation of NF-kappaB and posttranslational modifications of histone deacetylase in macrophages. *Am. J. Physiol. Lung Cell Mol. Physiol.* 291:L46-57, 2006.

[65] Werner SL, Barken D, Hoffmann A: Stimulus specificity of gene expression programs determined by temporal control of IKK activity. *Science.* 309:1857-61, 2005.

[66] Ford PA, Durham AL, Russell RE, et al: Treatment effects of low-dose theophylline combined with an inhaled corticosteroid in COPD. *Chest.* 137:1338-44, 2010.

[67] Shi Y, He B, Kuchenbecker KM, et al: Inhibition of Wnt-2 and galectin-3 synergistically destabilizes beta-catenin and induces apoptosis in human colorectal cancer cells. *Int. J. Cancer.* 121:1175-81, 2007.

[68] Zhang Y, Goss AM, Cohen ED, et al: A Gata6-Wnt pathway required for epithelial stem cell development and airway regeneration. *Nat. Genet.* 40:862-70, 2008.

[69] Reynolds SD, Zemke AC, Giangreco A, et al: Conditional stabilization of beta-catenin expands the pool of lung stem cells. *Stem Cells.* 26:1337-46, 2008.

[70] Johnson SM, Grosshans H, Shingara J, et al: RAS is regulated by the let-7 microRNA family. *Cell.* 120:635-47, 2005.

[71] Weiss GJ, Bemis LT, Nakajima E, et al: EGFR regulation by microRNA in lung cancer: correlation with clinical response and survival to gefitinib and EGFR expression in cell lines. *Ann. Oncol.* 19:1053-9, 2008.

[72] Kim H, Kwon YM, Kim JS, et al: Elevated mRNA levels of DNA methyltransferase-1 as an independent prognostic factor in primary nonsmall cell lung cancer. *Cancer.* 107:1042-9, 2006.

[73] Lujambio A, Esteller M: CpG island hypermethylation of tumor suppressor microRNAs in human cancer. *Cell Cycle.* 6:1455-9, 2007.

[74] Wu X, Piper-Hunter MG, Crawford M, et al: MicroRNAs in the pathogenesis of Lung Cancer. *J. Thorac. Oncol.* 4:1028-34, 2009.

[75] Skrzypski M, Dziadziuszko R, Jassem J: MicroRNA in lung cancer diagnostics and treatment. *Mutat. Res.* 717:25-31, 2011.

[76] Liu X, Sempere LF, Guo Y, et al: Involvement of microRNAs in lung cancer biology and therapy. *Transl. Res.* 157:200-8, 2011.

[77] Sempere LF: Integrating contextual miRNA and protein signatures for diagnostic and treatment decisions in cancer. *Expert Rev. Mol. Diagn.* 11:813-27, 2011.

[78] Melo SA, Esteller M: Dysregulation of microRNAs in cancer: playing with fire. *FEBS Lett.* 585:2087-99, 2011.

[79] Osada H, Takahashi T: let-7 and miR-17-92: small-sized major players in lung cancer development. *Cancer Sci.* 102:9-17, 2011.

[80] Paccez JD, Vasques GJ, Correa RG, et al: The receptor tyrosine kinase Axl is an essential regulator of prostate cancer proliferation and tumor growth and represents a new therapeutic target. *Oncogene,* 2012.

[81] Krutzfeldt J, Rajewsky N, Braich R, et al: Silencing of microRNAs in vivo with 'antagomirs'. *Nature.* 438:685-9, 2005.

[82] Johnson CD, Esquela-Kerscher A, Stefani G, et al: The let-7 microRNA represses cell proliferation pathways in human cells. *Cancer Res.* 67:7713-22, 2007.

[83] Takamizawa J, Konishi H, Yanagisawa K, et al: Reduced expression of the let-7 microRNAs in human lung cancers in association with shortened postoperative survival. *Cancer Res.* 64:3753-6, 2004.

[84] Yanaihara N, Caplen N, Bowman E, et al: Unique microRNA molecular profiles in lung cancer diagnosis and prognosis. *Cancer Cell.* 9:189-98, 2006.

[85] Rabinowits G, Gercel-Taylor C, Day JM, et al: Exosomal microRNA: a diagnostic marker for lung cancer. *Clin. Lung Cancer.* 10:42-6, 2009.

[86] Lebanony D, Benjamin H, Gilad S, et al: Diagnostic assay based on hsa-miR-205 expression distinguishes squamous from nonsquamous non-small-cell lung carcinoma. *J. Clin. Oncol.* 27:2030-7, 2009.

[87] Liu F, Killian JK, Yang M, et al: Epigenomic alterations and gene expression profiles in respiratory epithelia exposed to cigarette smoke condensate. *Oncogene.* 29:3650-64, 2010.

[88] Belinsky SA, Palmisano WA, Gilliland FD, et al: Aberrant promoter methylation in bronchial epithelium and sputum from current and former smokers. *Cancer Res.* 62:2370-7, 2002.

[89] Palmisano WA, Divine KK, Saccomanno G, et al: Predicting lung cancer by detecting aberrant promoter methylation in sputum. *Cancer Res.* 60:5954-8, 2000.

[90] Belinsky SA, Liechty KC, Gentry FD, et al: Promoter hypermethylation of multiple genes in sputum precedes lung cancer incidence in a high-risk cohort. *Cancer Res.* 66:3338-44, 2006.

[91] Hegi ME, Diserens AC, Gorlia T, et al: MGMT gene silencing and benefit from temozolomide in glioblastoma. *N. Engl. J. Med.* 352:997-1003, 2005.

[92] Ramirez JL, Rosell R, Taron M, et al: 14-3-3sigma methylation in pretreatment serum circulating DNA of cisplatin-plus-gemcitabine-treated advanced non-small-cell lung cancer patients predicts survival: The Spanish Lung Cancer Group. *J. Clin. Oncol.* 23:9105-12, 2005.

[93] Yu SL, Chen HY, Chang GC, et al: MicroRNA signature predicts survival and relapse in lung cancer. *Cancer Cell.* 13:48-57, 2008.

[94] Jones PA, Baylin SB: The epigenomics of cancer. *Cell.* 128:683-92, 2007.

[95] Digel W, Lubbert M: DNA methylation disturbances as novel therapeutic target in lung cancer: Preclinical and clinical results. *Critical Reviews in Oncology Hematology.* 55:1-11, 2005.

[96] Laird PW, Jackson-Grusby L, Fazeli A, et al: Suppression of intestinal neoplasia by DNA hypomethylation. *Cell.* 81:197-205, 1995.

[97] Cedar H, Bergman Y: Epigenetics of haematopoietic cell development. *Nat. Rev. Immunol.* 11:478-88, 2011.

[98] Weiss AJ, Stambaugh JE, Mastrangelo MJ, et al: Phase I study of 5-azacytidine (NSC-102816). *Cancer Chemother. Rep*. 56:413-9, 1972.

[99] Holoye PY, Dhingra HM, Umsawasdi T, et al: Phase II study of 5,6-dihydro-5-azacytidine in extensive, untreated non-small cell lung cancer. *Cancer Treat. Rep.* 71:859-60, 1987.

[100] Momparler RL, Ayoub J: Potential of 5-aza-2'-deoxycytidine (Decitabine) a potent inhibitor of DNA methylation for therapy of advanced non-small cell lung cancer. *Lung Cancer*. 34 Suppl 4:S111-5, 2001.

[101] Schrump DS, Fischette MR, Nguyen DM, et al: Phase I study of decitabine-mediated gene expression in patients with cancers involving the lungs, esophagus, or pleura. *Clin. Cancer Res.* 12:5777-85, 2006.

[102] Stewart DJ, Issa JP, Kurzrock R, et al: Decitabine effect on tumor global DNA methylation and other parameters in a phase I trial in refractory solid tumors and lymphomas. *Clin. Cancer Res.* 15:3881-8, 2009.

[103] Schwartsmann G, Schunemann H, Gorini CN, et al: A phase I trial of cisplatin plus decitabine, a new DNA-hypomethylating agent, in patients with advanced solid tumors and a follow-up early phase II evaluation in patients with inoperable non-small cell lung cancer. *Invest. New Drugs.* 18:83-91, 2000.

[104] Appleton K, Mackay HJ, Judson I, et al: Phase I and pharmacodynamic trial of the DNA methyltransferase inhibitor decitabine and carboplatin in solid tumors. *J. Clin. Oncol*. 25:4603-9, 2007.

[105] Bolden JE, Peart MJ, Johnstone RW: Anticancer activities of histone deacetylase inhibitors. *Nat. Rev. Drug Discov*. 5:769-84, 2006.

[106] Yoo CB, Jones PA: Epigenetic therapy of cancer: past, present and future. *Nat. Rev. Drug Discov*. 5:37-50, 2006.

[107] Minucci S, Pelicci PG: Histone deacetylase inhibitors and the promise of epigenetic (and more) treatments for cancer. *Nat. Rev. Cancer*. 6:38-51, 2006.

[108] Schrump DS: Cytotoxicity mediated by histone deacetylase inhibitors in cancer cells: mechanisms and potential clinical implications. *Clin. Cancer Res*. 15:3947-57, 2009.

[109] Ramalingam SS: Histone deacetylase inhibitors. *J. Thorac. Oncol.* 6:S1808-9, 2011.

[110] Olsen EA, Kim YH, Kuzel TM, et al: Phase IIb multicenter trial of vorinostat in patients with persistent, progressive, or treatment refractory cutaneous T-cell lymphoma. *J. Clin. Oncol.* 25:3109-15, 2007.

[111] Traynor AM, Dubey S, Eickhoff JC, et al: Vorinostat (NSC# 701852) in patients with relapsed non-small cell lung cancer: a Wisconsin Oncology Network phase II study. *J. Thorac. Oncol*. 4:522-6, 2009.

[112] Ramalingam SS, Parise RA, Ramanathan RK, et al: Phase I and pharmacokinetic study of vorinostat, a histone deacetylase inhibitor, in combination with carboplatin and paclitaxel for advanced solid malignancies. *Clin. Cancer Res.* 13:3605-10, 2007.

[113] Ramalingam SS, Maitland ML, Frankel P, et al: Carboplatin and Paclitaxel in combination with either vorinostat or placebo for first-line therapy of advanced non-small-cell lung cancer. *J. Clin. Oncol*. 28:56-62, 2010.

[114] Belani C RS, Kalemkerian G: Randomized, double-blind phase II/III study of first-line paclitaxel (P) plus carboplatin (C) in combination with vorinostat or placebo in patients with advanced non-small-cell lung cancer (NSCLC). *Eur. J. Cancer. Suppl.* 7:507, 2009.

[115] Schrump DS, Nguyen DM, Kunst TE, et al: Phase I study of sequential deoxyazacytidine/depsipeptide infusion in patients with malignancies involving lungs or pleura. *Clin. Lung Cancer*. 4:186-92, 2002.

[116] Otterson GA, Hodgson L, Pang H, et al: Phase II study of the histone deacetylase inhibitor Romidepsin in relapsed small cell lung cancer (Cancer and Leukemia Group B 30304). *J. Thorac. Oncol*. 5:1644-8, 2010.

[117] Zhang W, Peyton M, Xie Y, et al: Histone deacetylase inhibitor romidepsin enhances anti-tumor effect of erlotinib in non-small cell lung cancer (NSCLC) cell lines. *J. Thorac. Oncol.* 4:161-6, 2009.

[118] Schrump DS, Fischette MR, Nguyen DM, et al: Clinical and molecular responses in lung cancer patients receiving Romidepsin. *Clin. Cancer Res.* 14:188-98, 2008.

[119] Witta SE, Gemmill RM, Hirsch FR, et al: Restoring E-cadherin expression increases sensitivity to epidermal growth factor receptor inhibitors in lung cancer cell lines. *Cancer Res.* 66:944-50, 2006.

[120] Zhu WG, Otterson GA: The interaction of histone deacetylase inhibitors and DNA methyltransferase inhibitors in the treatment of human cancer cells. *Curr. Med. Chem. Anticancer. Agents*. 3:187-99, 2003.

[121] Cameron EE, Bachman KE, Myohanen S, et al: Synergy of demethylation and histone deacetylase inhibition in the re-expression of genes silenced in cancer. *Nat. Genet.* 21:103-7, 1999.

[122] Gottlicher M, Minucci S, Zhu P, et al: Valproic acid defines a novel class of HDAC inhibitors inducing differentiation of transformed cells. *EMBO J.* 20:6969-78, 2001.

[123] Scherpereel A, Berghmans T, Lafitte JJ, et al: Valproate-doxorubicin: promising therapy for progressing mesothelioma. A phase II study. *Eur. Respir. J.* 37:129-35, 2011.

[124] Chu BF, Karpenko MJ, Liu Z, Aimiuwu J, Villalona-Calero MA, Chan KK, et al. Phase I study of 5-aza-2'-deoxycytidine in combination with valproic acid in non-small-cell lung cancer. *Cancer chemotherapy and pharmacology.* 2012 Oct 9. [Epub ahead of print]

[125] Lin J, Gilbert J, Rudek MA, et al: A phase I dose-finding study of 5-azacytidine in combination with sodium phenylbutyrate in patients with refractory solid tumors. *Clin. Cancer Res.* 15:6241-9, 2009.

[126] Stathis A, Hotte SJ, Chen EX, et al: Phase I study of decitabine in combination with vorinostat in patients with advanced solid tumors and non-Hodgkin's lymphomas. *Clin. Cancer Res.* 17:1582-90, 2011.

[127] Candelaria M, Gallardo-Rincon D, Arce C, et al: A phase II study of epigenetic therapy with hydralazine and magnesium valproate to overcome chemotherapy resistance in refractory solid tumors. *Ann. Oncol.* 18:1529-38, 2007.

[128] Braiteh F, Soriano AO, Garcia-Manero G, et al: Phase I study of epigenetic modulation with 5-azacytidine and valproic acid in patients with advanced cancers. *Clin. Cancer Res.* 14:6296-301, 2008.

[129] Moving AHEAD with an international human epigenome project. *Nature*. 454:711-5, 2008.

In: Non-Small Cell Lung Cancer: New Research
Editor: Lina Pasquariello
ISBN: 978-1-62417-804-7

Chapter 4

Molecular Profiling in Lung Cancer Specimens Leads to Targeted Therapeutic Options in Patients with Non-Small Cell Lung Carcinoma (NSCLC)

Kirtee Raparia,[1] Peter Kulesza[1,*] and Melissa Johnson[2]
[1]Department of Pathology, Feinberg School of Medicine, Northwestern University, Chicago, IL, US
[2]Department of Medicine-Hematology/Oncology, Feinberg School of Medicine, Northwestern University, Chicago, IL, US

Abstract

After a period of stagnation in lung cancer therapeutics, a remarkable molecular revolution occurred in mid-2000's. Molecular characterization of lung carcinoma coincided with the development, and utilization of targeted therapeutic agents. The discovery of EGFR led the movement: after some false starts (INTACT1 and 2), small molecule tyrosine kinase inhibitors gefitinib and then erlotinib gained FDA-approval. Basic science hypotheses of oncogene addition and the discovery of activating mutations has rapidly transitioned from bench to bedside, resulting in a recommendation for up-front testing of lung cancer patients, and the use of targeted agents as first line therapy. Subsequent drug-target pairs followed, such as crizotinib-ALK-EML rearrangements, and in this case the clinical use approval was followed within days by a separate companion diagnostic, underscoring the need for rethinking of the regulatory review and approval paradigm. At this time, a queue of oncogene targets is forming, and inhibitors are being tested in clinical trials with some success: ROS1, RET, C-Met, and BRAF are among them, although others like KRAS remain difficult to target effectively. Regardless of the molecular target, lesional tissue is required for any analysis, and in this process the

* E-mail: p-kulesza@northwestern.edu.

diagnosis by a pathologist remains the primary step. The challenge arises as the low morbidity means of tissue procurement result in ever smaller amounts of material, while the numbers and variety of assay platforms necessary to match drugs to targets increases. Given this paradigm only a multiplexed approach is feasible, which consequently enforces a common assay platform. Mutational profiling, such as SNaPshot, which captures all known abnormalities should find its way into regular diagnostic practice, and be included in the planning of all lung cancer trials involving new targeted agents.

Introduction

Development of invasive lung carcinoma is a result of sequential accumulation of genetic and epigenetic changes that are also reflected in the morphology of these tumors. Remarkable advances in the understanding of NSCLC have been made on both a histologic and molecular basis. Lung cancer is now considered a heterogeneous group of diseases and mutational profiling is now becoming routine practice in thoracic oncology. With the discovery of activating mutations in the epidermal growth factor receptor (*EGFR*) of lung adenocarcinoma tumors, [1-3] and the subsequent recognition that this biomarker predicted high response rates and prolonged progression-free survival after treatment with *EGFR* tyrosine kinase inhibitors (TKIs), [4] clinical decision-making for lung cancer patients began a dramatic revolution. Prior to 2004, the tumors of all patients with metastatic non-small cell lung cancers (NSCLC) were presumed to be tobacco-related, all patients had marginal responses to platinum-based chemotherapies, and survived a median of eight months after diagnosis. [5] Nearly a decade later, medical oncologists and pathologists alike recognize NSCLC, in particular lung adenocarcinoma, to be composed of a number of histologic sub-types, associated with underlying genetic mutations. These oncogenes, including *EGFR*, are thought to determine, or "drive" adenocarcinoma development and tumor responses to therapy. The growing number of mutated oncogenes which contribute to adenocarcinoma tumorigenesis also explains the heterogeneous phenotypes and survival outcomes observed among patients who carry the same "lung cancer" diagnosis. As a result, a "personalized" method of selecting treatments have replaced the "one treatment fits all" approach—in which clinicians strive to identify oncogene targets within patient tumor tissue and match it with available small molecular inhibitors. Here, we review the identified oncogenes to date and the small molecule inhibitors currently prescribed to patients in clinical practice.

EGFR: The Prototype Oncogene

The most frequently targeted pathways in non-small cell carcinoma involve epidermal growth factor receptor. *EGFR (HER-1/ErbB1)* is a member of the *ErbB* family of tyrosine kinase receptors (TKs), which includes *HER-1/ErB1, HER-2/neu/ErB2, HER-3/ErB3,* and *HER-4/ErB4*. *EGFR* mutations are found in ~10% of patients with NSCLCs (reports range from 5 to 20% in Caucasians and 20 to 60% in Asian patients with adenocarcinomas). [6-9] Patients from different ethnic backgrounds with NSCLC exhibit several epidemiologic differences, including a higher proportion of nonsmoking women with tumors having *EGFR* activating somatic mutations, and clinical responses to tyrosine kinase inhibitor therapy in patients from East Asia. Although *EGFR* mutations are most frequently observed in never-smoker females with bronchioalveolar carcinomas (BAC) and invasive adenocarcinoma with predominant BAC component, a significant percentage of them have also been noted in acinar and papillary variants of adenocarcinoma. [2, 8, 10-12] Multiple approaches for assessment of *EGFR* status in lung carcinoma have been introduced including DNA mutational analysis, fluorescence *in situ* hybridization (FISH)/ chromogenic *in situ* hybridization (CISH) and immunohistochemistry. Sanger DNA direct sequencing is the most common mutational technique employed in most laboratories.

The Iressa Pan-Asia Study (IPASS) is recognized as the landmark trial which peaked the interest of clinicians and scientists alike about the predictive importance of activating mutations in *EGFR* (ie. exon 19 deletions or exon 21 L858R point mutations) for the treatment of lung adenocarcinoma. In this phase III trial, Mok et al. randomized untreated Asian non-smokers or former light-smokers with lung adenocarcinoma to receive small molecule EGFR TKI gefitinib versus standard chemotherapy (carboplatin and paclitaxel). [4] A prospectively-planned analysis of treatment efficacy based upon the presence of mutated *EGFR* confirmed that patients whose tumors harbored a mutation in *EGFR* had higher response rates (71.2% vs. 47.3%) and longer progression-free survival (PFS) (9.5 months vs. 6.3 months) when treated with gefitinib as compared with chemotherapy (hazard ratio for progression, 0.48; 95% CI,0.36 to 0.64; P<0.001). In contrast, patients whose tumors did not have mutations in *EGFR* had *shorter* PFS when treated with gefitinib as compared with carboplatin and paclitaxel (hazard ratio for progression, 2.85; 95% CI, 2.05 to 3.98; P<0.001). IPASS demonstrated "proof of principle" that the presence of an activating mutation in *EGFR* predicted tumor sensitivity to *EGFR*-targeted inhibitor gefitinib. Patients having the clinical characteristics previously associated with response to EGFR TKIs (i.e., Asian ethnicity, non-smoking status, adenocarcinoma tumor histology)[13], were therefore more likely to have *EGFR* mutations in their tumors.

Since IPASS was published, there have been several other studies confirming the impact of *EGFR* mutations on lung cancer treatment outcomes. Maemondo et al. randomized patients with *EGFR*-mutated tumors to receive gefitinib or chemotherapy (carboplatin and paclitaxel), and demonstrated higher response rates (74% vs. 31%) and longer PFS for patients treated with gefitinib (10.8 months vs. 5.4 months, hazard ratio 0.30; 95% CI, 0.22-0.41, p<0.001) (North-East Japan Study Group). [14] Mitsudomi et al. randomized patients with *EGFR*-mutated tumors to gefitinib or chemotherapy (cisplatin and docetaxel) with similar improvements in median PFS for patients treated with gefitinib (9.2 months vs. 6.3 months, hazard ratio 0.5; 95% CI, 0.34-0.71, p<0.0001) (WJTOG3405-West Japan Oncology Group). [15] The OPTIMAL study tested the same hypothesis using EGFR TKI erlotinib versus chemotherapy (carboplatin and gemcitabine) in Chinese patients, and demonstrated for the third time in Asian patients an improvement in median PFS for patients treated with erlotinib, nearly three times that of patients treated with chemotherapy (13.1 months vs. 4.6 months, hazard ratio 0.16; 95% CI, 0.10-0.26; P<0.001)). [16] Finally, Rosell et al. published the EURTAC trial, demonstrating that even among Caucasian patients where *EGFR* mutations are less common (only 10-20% of lung adenocarcinoma), those with *EGFR* mutations treated with erlotinib had improved PFS as compared to those treated with chemotherapy (cisplatin and docetaxel) (9.7 months vs. 5.2 months, HR 0.37; 95% CI, 0.25-0.54; p<0.0001). [17] Taken together, these studies demonstrated that the presence of activating *EGFR* mutations is associated with favorable responses to targeted agents gefitinib and erlotinib. The fact the results were replicated in both Asian and European patients, and with either gefitinib or erlotinib, was important, because it demonstrated that analysis of *EGFR* mutation status was feasible in all racial populations, and that all patients with *EGFR* mutations stand to gain from treatment with EGFR TKIs. As a result of these studies, the National Comprehensive Cancer Network (NCCN) and the American Society of Clinical Oncology (ASCO) amended United States practice guidelines to recommend upfront testing for *EGFR* be performed for all patients with a lung adenocarcinoma diagnosis to ensure that patients with *EGFR* mutations can be offered EGFR TKI rather than chemotherapy for first-line treatment. [2, 18]

EML4-ALK: Applying the "Driver" Oncogene Principle

EML4-ALK is an aberrant gene-fusion product caused by the translocation of the N-terminal portion of the EML4 gene with the tyrosine kinase domain of *ALK*, resulting in constitutive kinase activation of *ALK* and cancer development in 3-5% of patients with lung adenocarcinoma. [19] This second oncogenic driver mutation is more prevalent among younger male patients with little or no smoking history, and *ALK*-positive tumors exhibit adenocarcinoma histology with predominant signet-ring features. [20] Fluorescence *in situ* hybridization (FISH) has been regarded as a gold standard method for detecting *ALK* rearrangement.

However, a newly developed *ALK* chromogenic *in situ* hybridization (CISH), real time polymerase chain reaction and *ALK* protein expression by immunohistochemistry (IHC) has been also shown to be useful methods in determining *ALK* gene rearrangement. [21]

Patients with *ALK*-positive tumors were first treated with small molecule inhibitor crizotinib, designed to inhibit both *ALK* and *MET*, [22-23 in an expanded cohort in a phase I clinical trial of pre-treated patients with lung adenocarcinoma who harbored *EML4-ALK* translocations. *ALK*-positive patients were found to have higher response rates (61%) and longer progression-free survival (10 months) when treated with crizotinib as compared with historical controls who received conventional second line-chemotherapies (responses rates <10%, median PFS 3 months). [24-27] A second single-arm phase II study reported comparable response rates (50%) in 136 pre-treated lung adenocarcinoma patients with *EML4-ALK* fusions with responses lasting 12 months. [28]

Based on the results of these two early phase trials and one still on-going phase II trial (NCT00932451), regulatory leaders at the FDA granted an accelerated approval of crizotinib for the treatment of *ALK*-positive patients with lung adenocarcinoma in August 2011.

Quickly NCCN and ASCO recommended *EML4-ALK* testing be moved up front with *EGFR* to be tested among all new lung adenocarcinoma diagnoses. [2, 29]

Crizotinib gained its regulatory approval only four years after the pre-clinical discovery of *EML4-ALK*, [19] a remarkable feat in drug development compared with the national average for FDA approval of a new drug, 12 years. The FDA approval of crizotinib was made possible, in part, due to the "proof of principle" demonstrated by IPASS and other trials evaluating *EGFR*– careful molecular selection of patients being evaluated with a targeted inhibitor is crucial to demonstrate the efficacy of the novel agent. Crizotinib's approval also underscored a second changing paradigm within the lung cancer field that small molecular inhibitors should be tested in smaller molecularly select groups of patients, rather than the conventional phase III trial design enrolling large numbers of unselected populations.

Thus, the discovery of oncogene-driven lung adenocarcinoma has spurred not just revisions to the clinical approach to diagnosis and treatment of patients, but also adjustments to trial design and regulatory approval expectations for novel targeted therapies.

To date there have been no large, phase III trials evaluating crizotinib compared with chemotherapy (although two are on-going (NCT01154140 and NCT00932893). Clinical experience with this oncogene and inhibitor is less mature than that with *EGFR*, and the impact that crizotinib may have on extending survival outcomes for *ALK*-positive patients has not yet been clearly defined. In a retrospective analysis recently published, Shaw et al. reported the outcomes of *ALK*-positive patients treated with crizotinib, in addition to those of *ALK*-positive patients and *ALK*-negative controls treated with chemotherapy.

While not powered for true comparisons between patient cohorts, *ALK*-positive patients treated with second-line or third-line crizotinib had longer survival outcomes than *ALK*-positive patients treated with any second-line therapy (median overall survival not reached (NR) (95% CI, 14 months to NR) vs. 6 months (95% CI, 4-17) (hazard ratio 0.36, 95% CI 0.17-0.75, p=0.004). *ALK*-positive patients treated with chemotherapy lived similar amounts of time as wild-type lung cancer control patients (median overall survival 20 months (95% CI, 13-26) vs. 15 months (95% CI, 13-17), p=0.244). While retrospective and non-randomized, this analysis suggests that treatment with crizotinib may prolong survival outcomes for *ALK*-positive patients. [30] The two on-going phase III studies for ALK-positive patients, one comparing crizotinib with platinum chemotherapies and pemetrexed in the first-line setting, and another comparing crizotinib with either second-line docetaxel or pemetrexed in the second-line setting will hopefully provide more insight about this molecular sub-group of patients.

ROS1: New Oncogene, Established Inhibitor

The success of crizotinib has spurred interest in still other mutated oncogenes and the small molecule therapies which may inhibit them. *ROS1* is the most recent addition to the growing number of receptor tyrosine kinases implicated in lung cancer pathogenesis.

ROS1 is a member of the insulin receptor family that becomes constitutively activated after chromosomal translocation events. *ROS1* was first linked with lung cancer development after the activated kinase was identified in a NSCLC cell line (HCC78; *SLC34A2-ROS1*), and found also in a genetic screen of a tumor samples from lung cancer patients (*CD74-ROS1*) in 2007. [31]

Approximately 1.5 % of screened patients in one recently published report were identified as harboring chromosomal abnormalities involving *ROS1*, approximately half the prevalence of *EML4-ALK*. [32] Like patients with *EGFR* mutations or *ALK* translocations, patients harboring *ROS1* rearrangements are more likely to be Asian, younger at diagnosis and never-smokers, although the histopathologic features of the tumors of these patients may be more heterogeneous (ie., varying tumor grade, with some demonstrating poorly differentiated features with highly atypical infiltrating tumor cells was described in the first report of *ROS1*-mutated tumors) [32].

In pre-clinical experiments, HCC78 cell lines with *ROS1* mutations were sensitive to treatment with selective ALK inhibitor TAE684. [22] Based on this scientific finding, and applying the lessons learned from the *EGFR* and *EML4-ALK* investigations, the first never-smoker with multi-focal adenocarcinoma of the lung harboring a *ROS1* mutation was treated with crizotinib in April 2011. Rapidly his lung cancer-related symptoms improved and at 8 weeks, restaging scans showed near complete radiographic response, which lasted at least six months at the time the case report was published. [24, 32]

c-Met

Several studies have documented overexpression and/or amplification of *c-Met* in lung adenocarcinoma. Takanami *et al.* reported an association between *c-Met* overexpression and decreased patient survival. [33] Other studies reported *c-Met* expression in patients with higher pathological stage and lymph node metastasis.[34] The *c-Met* may be an alternative pathway to EGFR in the activation of AKT in lung adenocarcinomas, and thus may provide an alternative therapeutic approach in the patients with tumors displaying resistance to EGFR inhibitors.

The MET pathway can be inhibited by monoclonal antibodies against hepatocyte growth factor or those directed against a MET receptor, or by MET TKIs. A recent phase I trial with a human anti-hepatocyte growth factor monoclonal antibody, AMG102 in combination with bevacizumab in patients with solid tumors demonstrated inhibition of tumors in patients with lung cancer. [35] The anti-MET receptor monoclonal antibody, MetMab has been evaluated in a phase II trial in combination with erlotinib and the results suggest benefit in patients with overexpression of MET. [36] ARQ197 is a selective, non-ATP competitive inhibitor of MET kinase. Results showed that ARQ-197 is well-tolerated and prolongs PFS, however studies are still ongoing. [37]

KIF5B-RET Fusions

Whole-transcriptome sequencing studies performed by Kohno et al. reported a novel fusion between *KIF5B* (the kinesin family 5B gene) and the ret proto-oncogene (RET) gene, leading to an activation of RET kinase in lung adenocarcinomas. This is a new driver mutation present in 1–2% of lung adenocarcinoma in patients from Japan and United States. *KIF5B-RET* fusion was not seen in any of the squamous-cell carcinoma, large-cell carcinoma and small-cell lung carcinomas. This fusion gene may serve as a promising molecular target for the personalized therapy in a selected subset of patients with lung cancer.[38-39]

KRAS: Elusive Oncogene Target

There are a number of other mutations identified as oncogenic drivers that are proposed to be responsible for other molecular sub-groups of lung adenocarcinoma. The *ras* proteins or p21*ras* belong to the small guanosine triphosphatase (GTPase) superfamily, of which *KRAS*,

HRAS, and *NRAS* are the 3 best known among various members. *KRAS* accounts for most of the *ras* mutations found in the majority of human malignancies. Notably, *KRAS* accounts for 90% of *ras* mutations in lung adenocarcinomas. [40] A landmark study in 1984 demonstrated that a human lung cancer specimen has an activating *KRAS* mutation that was not found in corresponding normal tissue.[41] *KRAS* mutations are more frequently found in the tumors of patients with heavy tobacco exposure, but are also encountered among never-smokers with lung cancer. [42]

While the data is somewhat conflicting, patients whose tumors harbor *KRAS* mutations appear to have a shorter prognosis compared to patients with *EGFR* mutations, both in early stage as well as advanced lung cancer populations.[43-44] *KRAS* mutations also predict for tumors with primary resistance to treatment with EGFR TKIs. [40, 45]

However, efforts to identify *KRAS*-directed small molecule inhibitors have been unsuccessful, and few *KRAS*-targeted agents have been brought forward to be tested in human subjects on clinical trials. [46] One reason drug development has been unsuccessful may be that mutated *KRAS* proteins appear to lose their normal enzymatic function once they are constitutively activated. *Loss*-of-function mutations appear much more difficult to target with small molecular inhibitors as compared to *gain*-of-function mutations, such as *EGFR*, *EML4-ALK,* and *ROS1.* [40] Current efforts to target *KRAS*-driven lung adenocarcinoma involve inhibition of proteins downstream of *KRAS* in the *RAS/RAF/MEK* signal transduction pathway, for example, inhibition of *RAF* (sorafenib) [47] (NCT01248247) and inhibition of *MEK 1/2* (GSK1120212) (NCT01362296).

Additional trials are evaluating a combination approach for targeting *KRAS,* for example, inhibition of *c-MET* (ARQ-197) and *EGFR* (erlotinib) [48] (NCT01395758), or inhibition of *MEK* (AZD6244) and *EGFR* (erlotinib) (NCT01229150).

Vascular Endothelial Growth Factor (VEGF)

VEGF signaling pathway is an important target for novel antitumor therapies. VEGF plays a vital role in physiologic and pathologic angiogenesis, and it serves as a ligand for two receptors expressed on the surface of endothelial cells, *VEGFR-1 (FLT-1)* and *VEGFR-2 (KDR). VEGFR-2* plays a primary role in the activation of signaling pathways important in vascular permeability, endothelial cell proliferation, endothelial cell migration and cell survival. Angiogenesis is a key pathophysiologic event in tumor growth and survival. *VEGF* is strongly expressed in tumors in patients with NSCLC and correlates with increased microvascular density and poor clinical outcome.[49]

Bevacizumab is a monoclonal antibody that targets circulating VEGF and inhibits VEGF binding to VEGF receptor. The value of VEGF inhibition was initially established in a phase III trial (ECOG 4599), which included 878 previously untreated patients with advanced, nonsquamous NSCLC.[50] Patients with squamous cell carcinoma, brain metastasis, hemoptysis or having therapeutic anticoagulation were excluded to minimize the risk of pulmonary or intracerebral hemorrhage, based upon the results of the phase II study.[51] Patients receiving chemotherapy plus bevacizumab had significant increases in the objective response rate, overall survival, one- and two-year survival rates, and progression-free survival.

A second phase III randomized trial (AVAiL-Avastin in Lung Cancer) evaluated bevacizumab in combination with cisplatin and gemcitabine in 1043 patients.[52] This study revealed significant improvement in the primary endpoint (PFS), with the addition of bevacizumab compared with chemotherapy alone, at a median follow up of greater than 7 months.

New Oncogenes Seeking Inhibitors

Other mutated oncogene implicated in lung adenocarcinoma pathogenesis include *PIK3CA* [53], *BRAF* [54], *HER2*, [44, 55] *NRAS*, and *HRAS*. A novel fusion gene *KIF5B-RET* caused by a peri-centric inversion of chromosome 10, has recently been identified as another driver mutation in lung adenocarcinoma.[56-59] All of these newly-reported oncogene drivers occur in small percentages (i.e., 1-2% each) of all lung adenocarcinoma, and each sub-type defines a group of patients with diverse clinical characteristics. In contrast to *EGFR*, *EML4-ALK* and *KRAS*, which occur in lung adenocarcinoma, and in a mutually exclusive manner,[20, 45] *PIK3CA* has been reported in tumors of both adenocarcinoma and squamous cell histology, and are more likely to be co-expressed with other driver mutations such as *EGFR*, *KRAS* or *ALK*.[53] *BRAF* mutations have also been reported among both adenocarcinoma and squamous carcinoma of the lung. [54-55, 60] In distinction to *EGFR*, *EMLF-ALK* and *ROS1* mutations found more commonly among never-smokers with lung cancer, Paik et al. reported that patients with *BRAF* mutations were more common among current or former smokers. [54] A second report by Marchetti et al. found only patients with non-V600E BRAF mutations to be associated with lung cancer patients with smoking histories. [61]

Therapeutic Targets in Squamous Cell Carcinoma

Squamous cell carcinoma is the most prevalent subtype of lung cancer worldwide and its pathogenesis is linked to smoking and to lesser extent to other causes such as radiation, arsenic and chloromethyl ether exposure. Unlike the aforementioned advances in lung adenocarcinoma, the targeted and conventional therapeutics are poorly active in squamous cell carcinomas patients.

Drugs such as bevacizumab that inhibit VEGF are contraindicated in patients with squamous cell carcinoma due to increased risk of fatal hemorrhage. Bass et al showed that SOX2 is an amplified lineage-survival oncogene in lung squamous cell carcinoma.[62] Studies have confirmed recurrent amplification of SOX2 in up to 20% of squamous cell carcinoma patients. Weiss et al identified focal amplification of receptor tyrosine kinase fibroblast growth factor receptor 1 (FGFR1) in a subgroup of squamous-cell lung cancer patients, raising the possibility that FGFR inhibitors may be efficacious for this cohort of patients.[63] More recently, Hammerman et al identified a novel therapeutic target in up to 4% of squamous cell carcinoma patients. These patients harbored mutations in the discoidin domain receptor 2 (DDR2) tyrosine kinase gene. DDR2 is a receptor tyrosine kinase which signals in response to fibrillar collagen and promotes cell migration, proliferation and survival. The authors also found that treatment with the FDA approved src-abl inhibitor dasatinib, which has potent inhibitory activity on DDR2, effectively killed DDR2-mutant lung cancer cells.[64]

Role of the Pathologist in Resection and Small Biopsies/Cytology Specimens

Lung cancers are increasingly diagnosed and staged by transbronchial needle aspiration (TBNA), endobronchial ultrasound-guided TBNA (EBUS-TBNA) and endoscopic ultrasound-guided fine needle aspirations (EUS-FNA). [65-66]

There are several limiting factors in the diagnosis of NSCLC subtypes, which are magnified when tissue samples are small and limited. It is well established that poorly differentiated adenocarcinoma and squamous cell carcinoma can appear indistinguishable by routine light microscopy, particularly in small biopsies and cytology samples. In these small specimens and in poorly differentiated tumors, pathologists need to integrate morphology with immunohistochemistry, evaluating: thyroid transcription factor (TTF-1) and novel aspartic proteinase of the pepsin family (Napsin A) for adenocarcinoma and p63, p40 and cytokeratin 5/6 for squamous cell carcinoma; histochemical stains, *e.g.*, mucin staining for adenocarcinoma, and molecular studies to provide an appropriate diagnosis. [67-70] An immunohistochemical “cocktail” of adenocarcinoma and squamous cell carcinoma markers (nuclear and cytoplasmic marker combinations) can be performed on poorly differentiated tumors to improve the diagnostic subtyping and economizing the tissue for further molecular studies.

Although making the correct diagnosis on these small biopsies and cytological specimens is important, it is imperative that pathologists recognize the judicial use of the tissue to maximize the yield of molecular analysis from these specimens.

At times these biopsies are solely done for molecular studies; hence communication between the oncologist, pulmonologist, interventional radiologist, thoracic surgeon and pathologist is crucial.

Studies have shown that mutational analysis performed on the biopsies and cytological specimens is feasible and reliable, [66, 71] when compared with the histologic resection specimens from the same patients. [72]

The Future: Molecular Profiling

More research is necessary to understand these less common oncogene drivers, their corresponding tumor biology, and the best approach to comprehensive molecular analysis of all known oncogenes. As our understanding of the molecular complexity of lung carcinogenesis becomes more sophisticated, it will be nearly impossible to predict which mutated oncogene (or oncogenes) a particular patient may have based on clinical characteristics.

In some cases, patients already defy the convention clinical identifiers associated with *EGFR* tumors, for example, according to one report that 6% (95% CI, 4-9%) of current smokers and 15% (95% CI, 13-17%) of former smokers and 19% of men (95% CI, 16-22%) harbor *EGFR* mutations, [30] and another that African-American patients with lung adenocarcinoma harbor *EGFR* mutations in their lung adenocarcinoma tumors at similar frequencies to Caucasian patients. [73] These data underscore the importance of testing *all patients* with lung adenocarcinoma for mutated oncogenes. Medical oncologists will rely increasingly on the molecular analyses performed after diagnosis of lung adenocarcinoma to understand the molecular features which exist in a patient's tumor and select first-line treatments. Concerns over cost-effective testing have dictated the sequential analysis of one mutation at a time at some institutions. [74] However, individual tumor testing in this step-wise manner is not time-efficient, and may exhaust available tumor tissue before the correct mutation or mutations are identified.

An alternative approach to molecular analysis is comprehensive molecular profiling, such as the SNaPshot platform, a multiplexed PCR- based assay, which allows analysis of all mutations simultaneously and with much less tumor tissue and expense. [75] This approach to molecular analysis ensures that all mutations present in an individual patient's tumor tissue will be simultaneously identified, in contrast to a gradational approach where co-existing mutations might be over-looked. Sequist et al. reported the clinical utility of the SNaPShot platform in real-time clinical practice, with a median turn-around time of 2.8 weeks, thereby allowing oncologists to incorporate the pathologic information obtained from the analysis into first-line treatment selections.

As many as 51% of patients whose tumors were screened for driver mutations in this program (primarily caucasian patients with smoking histories) were found to harbor some mutation identified using SNaPshot. A second approach to a multiplex platform has been reported by the Lung Cancer Mutation Consortium, a collaboration of 14 different institutions which recently reported their efforts to genotype 1,000 lung adenocarcinomas for the presence of molecular driver mutations. Once again, the majority of patients included (54%) were found to harbor a mutation in their lung adenocarcinoma tumors, and were subsequently enrolled in a clinical trial testing an appropriate targeted inhibitor of the mutation identified. [76] Molecular profiling can therefore be viewed as a feasible approach to molecular analysis that will ensure timely, accurate therapy selections.

In conclusion, in the era of "personalized" therapies for lung cancer, we know that more than 50% of patients with lung adenocarcinoma are caused by mutated oncogenes. Extrapolating from lessons learned first from EGFR and subsequently from ALK, we understand that the genetic mutations underlying lung adenocarcinoma development are heterogeneous, and predict response to treatment with small molecule inhibitors. Medical oncologists require time-efficient identification of underlying driver mutations in order to select first-line treatments for their lung cancer patients. Future clinical investigations of novel small molecule inhibitors require enrollment be restricted to appropriate molecular sub-sets of patients with lung adenocarcinoma. Finally, extending the survival outcomes of all lung cancer patients beyond that possible with chemotherapy alone requires collaboration and communication between oncologists and pathologists to identify additional mutated oncogenes which may direct therapy for not only first-line treatments decisions, but for second-line and third-line treatments as well.

References

[1] Pao W, Miller V, Zakowski M, et al. EGF receptor gene mutations are common in lung cancers from "never smokers" and are associated with sensitivity of tumors to gefitinib and erlotinib. *Proc. Natl. Acad. Sci. U S A.* Sep. 7 2004; 101 (36):13306-13311.

[2] Lynch TJ, Bell DW, Sordella R, et al. Activating mutations in the epidermal growth factor receptor underlying responsiveness of non-small-cell lung cancer to gefitinib. *N. Engl. J. Med.* May 20 2004; 350 (21): 2129-2139.

[3] Paez JG, Janne PA, Lee JC, et al. EGFR mutations in lung cancer: correlation with clinical response to gefitinib therapy. *Science.* Jun. 4 2004; 304 (5676):1497-1500.

[4] Mok TS, Wu YL, Thongprasert S, et al. Gefitinib or carboplatin-paclitaxel in pulmonary adenocarcinoma. *N. Engl. J. Med.* Sep. 3 2009; 361 (10):947-957.

[5] Schiller JH, Harrington D, Belani CP, et al. Comparison of four chemotherapy regimens for advanced non-small-cell lung cancer. *N. Engl. J. Med.* Jan. 10 2002; 346 (2):92-98.

[6] Pao W, Girard N. New driver mutations in non-small-cell lung cancer. *Lancet Oncol.* Feb. 2011;12(2):175-180.

[7] Sequist LV, Bell DW, Lynch TJ, Haber DA. Molecular predictors of response to epidermal growth factor receptor antagonists in non-small-cell lung cancer. *J. Clin. Oncol.* Feb. 10 2007;25(5):587-595.

[8] Tokumo M, Toyooka S, Kiura K, et al. The relationship between epidermal growth factor receptor mutations and clinicopathologic features in non-small cell lung cancers. *Clinical cancer research : an official journal of the American Association for Cancer Research.* Feb. 1 2005;11(3):1167-1173.

[9] Li C, Sun Y, Fang Z, et al. Comprehensive analysis of epidermal growth factor receptor gene status in lung adenocarcinoma. *J. Thorac. Oncol.* Jun. 2011;6(6):1016-1021.

[10] Sun PL, Seol H, Lee HJ, et al. High Incidence of EGFR Mutations in Korean Men Smokers with No Intratumoral Heterogeneity of Lung Adenocarcinomas: Correlation with Histologic Subtypes, EGFR/TTF-1 Expressions, and Clinical Features. *J. Thorac. Oncol.* Feb. 2012; 7 (2): 323-330.

[11] Kosaka T, Yatabe Y, Endoh H, Kuwano H, Takahashi T, Mitsudomi T. Mutations of the epidermal growth factor receptor gene in lung cancer: biological and clinical implications. *Cancer Res.* Dec. 15 2004; 64(24):8919-8923.

[12] Leary AF, Castro DG, Nicholson AG, et al. Establishing an EGFR mutation screening service for non-small cell lung cancer - sample quality criteria and candidate histological predictors. *Eur. J. Cancer.* Jan. 2012;48(1):61-67.

[13] Shigematsu H, Lin L, Takahashi T, et al. Clinical and biological features associated with epidermal growth factor receptor gene mutations in lung cancers. *J. Natl. Cancer Inst.* Mar. 2 2005;97(5):339-346.

[14] Maemondo M, Inoue A, Kobayashi K, et al. Gefitinib or chemotherapy for non-small-cell lung cancer with mutated EGFR. *N. Engl. J. Med.* Jun. 24 2010;362(25):2380-2388.

[15] Mitsudomi T, Morita S, Yatabe Y, et al. Gefitinib versus cisplatin plus docetaxel in patients with non-small-cell lung cancer harbouring mutations of the epidermal growth

factor receptor (WJTOG3405): an open label, randomised phase 3 trial. *Lancet Oncol.* Feb. 2010;11(2):121-128.

[16] Zhou C, Wu YL, Chen G, et al. Erlotinib versus chemotherapy as first-line treatment for patients with advanced EGFR mutation-positive non-small-cell lung cancer (OPTIMAL, CTONG-0802): a multicentre, open-label, randomised, phase 3 study. *Lancet Oncol.* Aug. 2011;12(8):735-742.

[17] Rosell R, Carcereny E, Gervais R, et al. Erlotinib versus standard chemotherapy as first-line treatment for European patients with advanced EGFR mutation-positive non-small-cell lung cancer (EURTAC): a multicentre, open-label, randomised phase 3 trial. *Lancet Oncol.* Mar. 2012;13(3):239-246.

[18] Keedy VL, Temin S, Somerfield MR, et al. American Society of Clinical Oncology provisional clinical opinion: epidermal growth factor receptor (EGFR) Mutation testing for patients with advanced non-small-cell lung cancer considering first-line EGFR tyrosine kinase inhibitor therapy. *J. Clin. Oncol.* May 20 2011;29(15):2121-2127.

[19] Soda M, Choi YL, Enomoto M, et al. Identification of the transforming EML4-ALK fusion gene in non-small-cell lung cancer. *Nature.* Aug. 2 2007;448(7153):561-566.

[20] Shaw AT, Yeap BY, Mino-Kenudson M, et al. Clinical features and outcome of patients with non-small-cell lung cancer who harbor EML4-ALK. *J. Clin. Oncol.* Sep. 10 2009;27(26):4247-4253.

[21] Kim H, Yoo SB, Choe JY, et al. Detection of ALK gene rearrangement in non-small cell lung cancer: a comparison of fluorescence in situ hybridization and chromogenic in situ hybridization with correlation of ALK protein expression. *J. Thorac. Oncol.* Aug. 2011;6(8):1359-1366.

[22] McDermott U, Iafrate AJ, Gray NS, et al. Genomic alterations of anaplastic lymphoma kinase may sensitize tumors to anaplastic lymphoma kinase inhibitors. *Cancer Res.* May 1 2008;68(9):3389-3395.

[23] Christensen JG, Zou HY, Arango ME, et al. Cytoreductive antitumor activity of PF-2341066, a novel inhibitor of anaplastic lymphoma kinase and c-Met, in experimental models of anaplastic large-cell lymphoma. *Mol. Cancer Ther.* Dec. 2007;6(12):3314-3322.

[24] Kwak EL, Bang YJ, Camidge DR, et al. Anaplastic lymphoma kinase inhibition in non-small-cell lung cancer. *N. Engl. J. Med.* Oct. 28 2010; 363(18):1693-1703.

[25] Shepherd FA, Rodrigues Pereira J, Ciuleanu T, et al. Erlotinib in previously treated non-small-cell lung cancer. *N. Engl. J. Med.* Jul. 14 2005; 353(2):123-132.

[26] Hanna N, Shepherd FA, Fossella FV, et al. Randomized phase III trial of pemetrexed versus docetaxel in patients with non-small-cell lung cancer previously treated with chemotherapy. *J. Clin. Oncol.* May 1 2004; 22(9):1589-1597.

[27] Camidge DR BY-J, Kwak EL, et al. Progression-free survival (PFS) from a phase I study of crizotinib (PF-02341966) in patients with ALK-positive non-small cell lung cancer (NSCLC). *Proc. Am. Soc. Clin. Oncol.* 2011;29.

[28] Crino L KD, Riely GJ, et al. Initial phase II results with crizotinib in advanced ALK-positive non-small cell lung cancer (NSCLC): PROFILE 1005. *J. Clin. Oncol.* 2011;29 ((suppl; abstr 7514)).

[29] Vogelzang NJ, Benowitz SI, Adams S, et al. Clinical cancer advances 2011: Annual Report on Progress Against Cancer from the American Society of Clinical Oncology. *J. Clin. Oncol.* Jan. 1 2012;30(1):88-109.

[30] Shaw AT, Yeap BY, Solomon BJ, et al. Effect of crizotinib on overall survival in patients with advanced non-small-cell lung cancer harbouring ALK gene rearrangement: a retrospective analysis. *Lancet Oncol.* Oct. 2011;12(11):1004-1012.

[31] Rikova K, Guo A, Zeng Q, et al. Global survey of phosphotyrosine signaling identifies oncogenic kinases in lung cancer. *Cell.* Dec. 14 2007; 131(6):1190-1203.

[32] Bergethon K, Shaw AT, Ignatius Ou SH, et al. ROS1 Rearrangements Define a Unique Molecular Class of Lung Cancers. *J. Clin. Oncol.* Mar. 10 2012;30(8):863-870.

[33] Takanami I, Tanana F, Hashizume T, et al. Hepatocyte growth factor and c-Met/hepatocyte growth factor receptor in pulmonary adenocarcinomas: an evaluation of their expression as prognostic markers. *Oncology.* Sep.-Oct. 1996;53(5):392-397.

[34] Nakamura Y, Niki T, Goto A, et al. c-Met activation in lung adenocarcinoma tissues: an immunohistochemical analysis. *Cancer Sci.* Jul. 2007;98(7):1006-1013.

[35] Rosen PJ, Sweeney CJ, Park DJ, et al. A phase Ib study of AMG 102 in combination with bevacizumab or motesanib in patients with advanced solid tumors. *Clinical cancer research : an official journal of the American Association for Cancer Research.* May 1 2010; 16 (9): 2677-2687.

[36] Spigel DR ET, Ramlau R, et al. . Final efficacy results from OAM4558g, a randomized phase II study evaluating MetMAb or placebo in combination with erlotinib in advanced NSCLC. *J. Clin. Oncol.* 2011;29 (suppl; abstr 7505). Paper presented at: ASCO2011.

[37] Schiller J AA, Brugger D et al. Results from ARQ 197-209: A global randomized placebo-controlled phase II clinical trial of erlotinib plus ARQ 197 versus erlotinib plus placebo in previously treated EGFR inhibitor-naive patients with locally advanced or metastatic non-small cell lung cancer (NSCLC). *J. Clin. Oncol.* 28:18s, 2010 (suppl; abstr LBA7502). Paper presented at: ASCO2010.

[38] Kohno T, Ichikawa H, Totoki Y, et al. KIF5B-RET fusions in lung adenocarcinoma. *Nat. Med.* Mar. 2012;18(3):375-377.

[39] Ju YS, Lee WC, Shin JY, et al. A transforming KIF5B and RET gene fusion in lung adenocarcinoma revealed from whole-genome and transcriptome sequencing. *Genome Res.* Mar. 2012; 22 (3):436-445.

[40] Riely GJ, Marks J, Pao W. KRAS mutations in non-small cell lung cancer. *Proc. Am. Thorac. Soc.* Apr. 15 2009;6(2):201-205.

[41] Santos E, Martin-Zanca D, Reddy EP, Pierotti MA, Della Porta G, Barbacid M. Malignant activation of a K-ras oncogene in lung carcinoma but not in normal tissue of the same patient. *Science.* Feb. 17 1984; 223 (4637):661-664.

[42] Riely GJ, Kris MG, Rosenbaum D, et al. Frequency and distinctive spectrum of KRAS mutations in never smokers with lung adenocarcinoma. *Clin. Cancer Res.* Sep. 15 2008; 14 (18):5731-5734.

[43] Marks JL, Broderick S, Zhou Q, et al. Prognostic and therapeutic implications of EGFR and KRAS mutations in resected lung adenocarcinoma. *J. Thorac. Oncol.* Feb. 2008; 3 (2):111-116.

[44] Johnson ML SC, Paik PK, Janjigian YY, Pao W, Kris MG, Ladanyi M, Riely GJ. Association of KRAS and EGFR mutations with survival in patients with advanced lung adenocarcinoma. *J. Clin. Oncol.* 2010; 28 (suppl; abstr 7541).

[45] Pao W, Wang TY, Riely GJ, et al. KRAS mutations and primary resistance of lung adenocarcinomas to gefitinib or erlotinib. *PLoS Med.* Jan. 2005; 2 (1):e17.

[46] Riely GJ, Johnson ML, Medina C, et al. A phase II trial of Salirasib in patients with lung adenocarcinomas with KRAS mutations. *J. Thorac. Oncol.* Aug. 2011; 6 (8):1435-1437.

[47] Kim ES HR, Wistuba II, Lee JJ, Blumenschein GR, Tsao A, Stewart DJ, Hicks ME, Erasmus J, Gupta S, Alden CM, Liu S, Tang X, Khuri FR, Tran HT, Johnson BE, Heymach JV, Mao L, Fossella F, Kies MS, Papadimitrakopoulou V, Davis SE, Lippman SM, Wong WK. The BATTLE Trial: Personalizing Therapy for Lung Cancer. *Cancer Discovery.* 2011; 1 (1):44-53.

[48] Sequist LV, von Pawel J, Garmey EG, et al. Randomized phase II study of erlotinib plus tivantinib versus erlotinib plus placebo in previously treated non-small-cell lung cancer. *J. Clin. Oncol.* Aug. 20 2011; 29 (24): 3307-3315.

[49] O'Byrne KJ, Koukourakis MI, Giatromanolaki A, et al. Vascular endothelial growth factor, platelet-derived endothelial cell growth factor and angiogenesis in non-small-cell lung cancer. *Br. J. Cancer.* Apr. 2000; 82 (8):1427-1432.

[50] Sandler A, Gray R, Perry MC, et al. Paclitaxel-carboplatin alone or with bevacizumab for non-small-cell lung cancer. *N. Engl. J. Med.* Dec. 14 2006; 355 (24):2542-2550.

[51] Johnson DH, Fehrenbacher L, Novotny WF, et al. Randomized phase II trial comparing bevacizumab plus carboplatin and paclitaxel with carboplatin and paclitaxel alone in previously untreated locally advanced or metastatic non-small-cell lung cancer. *J. Clin. Oncol.* Jun. 1 2004; 22 (11): 2184-2191.

[52] Reck M, von Pawel J, Zatloukal P, et al. Overall survival with cisplatin-gemcitabine and bevacizumab or placebo as first-line therapy for nonsquamous non-small-cell lung cancer: results from a randomised phase III trial (AVAiL). *Ann. Oncol.* Sep. 2010; 21 (9):1804-1809.

[53] Chaft JE, Arcila ME, Paik PK, et al. Coexistence of PIK3CA and other oncogene mutations in lung adenocarcinoma-rationale for comprehensive mutation profiling. *Clin. Cancer Res.* Feb. 2012;11 (2): 485-491.

[54] Paik PK, Arcila ME, Fara M, et al. Clinical characteristics of patients with lung adenocarcinomas harboring BRAF mutations. *J. Clin. Oncol.* May 20 2011;29(15):2046-2051.

[55] Arcila ME CJ, Nafa K, Kris MG, Zakowski MF, Ladanyi M. Molecular and clinicopathologic characteristics of HER2-mutant lung adenocarcinoma. *Proc. Am. Soc. Clin. Oncol.* 2011;29 (suppl; abstr. 10596).

[56] Kohno T, Ichikawa H, Totoki Y, et al. KIF5B-RET fusions in lung adenocarcinoma. *Nature Medicine.* Mar. 2012; 18 (3):375-377.

[57] Ju YS, Lee WC, Shin JY, et al. A transforming KIF5B and RET gene fusion in lung adenocarcinoma revealed from whole-genome and transcriptome sequencing. *Genome Research.* Mar. 2012; 22 (3): 436-445.

[58] Lipson D, Capelletti M, Yelensky R, et al. Identification of new ALK and RET gene fusions from colorectal and lung cancer biopsies. *Nature Medicine.* Mar. 2012; 18 (3):382-384.

[59] Takeuchi K, Soda M, Togashi Y, et al. RET, ROS1 and ALK fusions in lung cancer. *Nature Medicine.* Mar. 2012;18(3):378-381.

[60] Pratilas CA, Hanrahan AJ, Halilovic E, et al. Genetic predictors of MEK dependence in non-small cell lung cancer. *Cancer Res.* Nov 15 2008; 68 (22): 9375-9383.

[61] Marchetti A, Felicioni L, Malatesta S, et al. Clinical features and outcome of patients with non-small-cell lung cancer harboring BRAF mutations. *J. Clin. Oncol.* Sep. 10 2011; 29 (26): 3574-3579.

[62] Bass AJ, Watanabe H, Mermel CH, et al. SOX2 is an amplified lineage-survival oncogene in lung and esophageal squamous cell carcinomas. *Nat. Genet.* Nov. 2009; 41 (11):1238-1242.

[63] Weiss J, Sos ML, Seidel D, et al. Frequent and focal FGFR1 amplification associates with therapeutically tractable FGFR1 dependency in squamous cell lung cancer. *Sci. Transl. Med.* Dec. 15 2010;2(62):62ra93.

[64] Hammerman PS, Sos ML, Ramos AH, et al. Mutations in the DDR2 kinase gene identify a novel therapeutic target in squamous cell lung cancer. *Cancer Discov.* Apr. 3 2011;1(1):78-89.

[65] Shah PL, Singh S, Bower M, Livni N, Padley S, Nicholson AG. The role of transbronchial fine needle aspiration in an integrated care pathway for the assessment of patients with suspected lung cancer. *J. Thorac. Oncol.* May 2006;1(4):324-327.

[66] Santis G, Angell R, Nickless G, et al. Screening for EGFR and KRAS mutations in endobronchial ultrasound derived transbronchial needle aspirates in non-small cell lung cancer using COLD-PCR. *PLoS One.* 2011; 6(9): e25191.

[67] Travis WD, Rekhtman N. Pathological diagnosis and classification of lung cancer in small biopsies and cytology: strategic management of tissue for molecular testing. *Semin. Respir. Crit. Care Med.* Feb. 2011; 32 (1): 22-31.

[68] Travis WD, Rekhtman N, Riley GJ, et al. Pathologic diagnosis of advanced lung cancer based on small biopsies and cytology: a paradigm shift. *J. Thorac. Oncol.* Apr. 2010; 5(4): 411-414.

[69] Bishop JA, Teruya-Feldstein J, Westra WH, Pelosi G, Travis WD, Rekhtman N. p40 (DeltaNp63) is superior to p63 for the diagnosis of pulmonary squamous cell carcinoma. *Mod. Pathol.* Nov. 4 2011.

[70] Mukhopadhyay S, Katzenstein AL. Subclassification of non-small cell lung carcinomas lacking morphologic differentiation on biopsy specimens: Utility of an immunohistochemical panel containing TTF-1, napsin A, p63, and CK5/6. *Am. J. Surg. Pathol.* Jan. 2011; 35 (1):15-25.

[71] Lozano MD, Zulueta JJ, Echeveste JI, et al. Assessment of epidermal growth factor receptor and K-ras mutation status in cytological stained smears of non-small cell lung cancer patients: correlation with clinical outcomes. *Oncologist.* 2011; 16 (6):877-885.

[72] Bruno P, Mariotta S, Ricci A, et al. Reliability of Direct Sequencing of EGFR: Comparison between Cytological and Histological Samples from the Same Patient. *Anticancer Res.* Dec. 2011; 31 (12): 4207-4210.

[73] Reinersman JM, Johnson ML, Riely GJ, et al. Frequency of EGFR and KRAS mutations in lung adenocarcinomas in African Americans. *J. Thorac. Oncol.* Jan. 2011; 6 (1):28-31.

[74] Bunn PA, Jr., Doebele RC. Genetic testing for lung cancer: reflex versus clinical selection. *J. Clin. Oncol.* May 20 2011; 29 (15):1943-1945.

[75] Sequist LV, Heist RS, Shaw AT, et al. Implementing multiplexed genotyping of non-small-cell lung cancers into routine clinical practice. *Ann. Oncol.* Dec. 2011; 22 (12):2616-2624.

[76] Kris MG JB, Kwiatkowski et al. Identification of driver mutations in tumor specimens from 1,000 patients with lung adenocarcinoma: The NCI's Lung Cancer Mutation Consortium (LCMC). *J. Clin. Oncol.* 2011; 29 ((suppl; abstr CRA7506)).

In: Non-Small Cell Lung Cancer: New Research
Editor: Lina Pasquariello

ISBN: 978-1-62417-804-7

Chapter 5

The Role of Radiation Dose Escalation in the Treatment of Stage III Locally Advanced Inoperable Non-Small Cell Lung Cancer: Where Are We Now?

Sudha Amarnath and Shilpen Patel
Department of Radiation Oncology, Fred Hutchinson Cancer Research Center, University of Washington, Seattle, WA, US

Abstract

Lung cancer is the leading cause of cancer mortality in both men and women. The majority of these patients present with non-small cell lung cancer (85%) and approximately 45% have locally advanced, stage III disease. Until the 1990s, radiation therapy alone was considered the standard treatment for patients with locally advanced, unresectable disease with median survival times of 10-12 months and 5-year survival rates of 5%. In the early 1990s, several randomized clinical trials showed a survival benefit when platinum-based chemotherapy was delivered concurrently with radiation therapy (RT), with median survival times of 16-17 months and 5-year survival rates of 20-30%. Concurrent chemo-radiation therapy thus became the new standard of care for patients with unresectable stage III disease.

Despite the improved survival outcomes, loco-regional recurrences still remain a problem. Based on radiation oncology first principles, it is felt that higher doses of radiation (up to 100 Gy) may be necessary to adequately control non-small cell lung cancers. Historically, however, doses of radiation therapy had been limited to approximately 60 Gy due to normal tissue dose tolerances and the risks of toxicities to the lung and surrounding tissues. With more modern radiation therapy techniques, such as intensity modulated radiation therapy (IMRT), the incorporation of PET, and 4-D CT treatment planning scans, the role of dose escalation to further improve survival and local control outcomes is being actively evaluated.

Several trials, including the phase I RTOG 0117 study found that higher doses of radiation (up to 74 Gy) could be safely tolerated with concurrent carboplatin and paclitaxel chemotherapy. A follow-up Phase II study demonstrated a survival benefit with this regimen with a median survival time of 21.6 months. Based on these promising results, a randomized phase III trial, RTOG 0617, was initiated comparing carboplatin and paclitaxel chemotherapy with concurrent RT to either 60 Gy or 74 Gy. The interim results of this study were presented at ASTRO 2011 and revealed no survival benefit in the higher dose arm despite similar toxicity profiles between the two groups. These surprising results warrant further evaluation. One hypothesis for the lack of survival benefit is that carboplatin and paclitaxel may represent a suboptimal chemotherapy doublet and that outcomes may be improved if cisplatin-based chemotherapy is given concurrently with increasing doses of radiation therapy. This combination has not yet been tested in clinical trials and is the basis of a current phase I trial at the University of Washington.

Introduction

Lung cancer is the leading cause of cancer death in both men and women worldwide. In the United States, it is the second most common type of cancer with an estimated 221,130 new diagnoses and 157,000 deaths in 2011.[1] Approximately 85% of lung cancers are of the non-small cell (NSCLC) type, which includes predominantly squamous and adenocarcinoma histologies.

The treatment paradigm for treating NSCLC varies by stage, with primary surgery considered the gold standard treatment for localized stage I and II tumors and chemotherapy typically the treatment of choice for stage IV widely metastatic disease. Approximately 45% of patients will present with stage IIIA/B disease. Stage III NSCLC consists of a wide spectrum of disease from extensively invasive primary tumors to low or high volume regional nodal disease or both. Although some stage IIIA tumors may be amenable to surgical resection, the vast majority of stage IIIA and IIIB tumors will be unresectable and must be treated with other modalities, typically a combination of radiation therapy and chemotherapy. Despite significant advances in treatment technology and supportive care, only moderate improvements in survival have been made over the last 20 years and the prognosis for these patients remains grim. In this article, we present a historical perspective on the treatment of locally advanced, unresectable stage III non small cell lung cancers and discuss current research that attempts to push the current boundaries of treatment with a goal of improving outcomes in these patients.

Treatment with Radiation Therapy Alone

Radiation therapy alone for the treatment of locally advanced bulky disease was first established by the Veterans Administration Lung Group study, published in 1968.[2] In this study, 800 patients were randomized to either chemotherapy alone, radiation therapy alone, or placebo. Patients were treated to 40-50 Gy, although due to technical limitations, one-third of patients received less than 40 Gy. Despite no significant differences in median overall survival between the radiation and placebo groups, there was a statistically significant difference in survival when the top 25% of long-term survivors in each group were evaluated. This subset analysis revealed an overall survival of 10.1 months in patients treated with radiation compared to 7.6 months in the placebo-treated arm.

This initial work led to the Radiation Therapy Oncology Group (RTOG) 73-01 study[3] that developed the standard of care for the treatment of stage III tumors until the 1990s. In this study, 447 patients with unresectable stage III tumors were placed into two different treatment protocol groups based on extent of disease: (1) less advanced tumors, including T1-T3, N0-N2 and (2) more advanced tumors, including T4 with any N-stage or patients with N3 disease. The patients in group 1 were randomized to varying doses of RT: 40 Gy split course (4 Gy/fx with 2 week break after 20 Gy), 40 Gy continuous (2 Gy/fx), 50 Gy continuous (2 Gy/fx), or 60 Gy continuous (2 Gy/fx). Group 2 patients were treated to lower doses due to technical limitations and will not be discussed here. Treatment volumes included the tumor, mediastinal and hilar lymph nodes with a spinal cord block. Initial results published in 1980 established 60 Gy in 2 Gy fractions to be the optimal dose as it was well-tolerated and led to improved freedom from progression with modest improvements in local control and survival. Unfortunately, the local control benefit was not durable and the benefit was lost after 2 years. With this regimen, median survival was 10 months and 5-year survival 5%. Patterns of failure analysis of this study group published in 1987 revealed an intrathoracic failure rate of 27% in the group 1 patients treated to 60 Gy, but an incidence of distant metastases of 75-80% leading the authors to conclude that higher radiation doses were necessary for improved local control and systemic therapy was necessary for improved survival.[4]

Concurrent Chemoradiation Therapy as the New Standard

Based on the poor local control and high rates of distant metastases seen with radiation therapy alone, several prospective randomized controlled trials in the 1980s and 1990s attempted to improve outcomes by combining chemotherapy and radiation therapy. CALGB 8433 was the first study to demonstrate a benefit to combining chemotherapy with radiation therapy. In this study conducted between 1984-1987, 155 patients with stage III disease were randomized to induction chemotherapy with cisplatin and vinblastine followed by 60 Gy RT versus 60 Gy RT alone. A significant improvement was seen in median survival and 5-year survival rates when radiation was given after induction chemotherapy (13.7 months and 19%) compared to radiotherapy alone (9.6 months and 7%). [5]

Kubota et. al. further demonstrated the importance of radiation therapy in improving local control and overall survival in combined modality treatment of locally advanced NSCLC.[6]

In that study, patients who responded to chemotherapy were randomized to radiotherapy versus no radiotherapy. Patients in the radiotherapy group had a 69% local control rate compared to only 6% in those who did not receive radiotherapy.

Furthermore, the 3-year overall survival rate increased from 3% to 29% with the addition of radiation. These results underscore the fact that radiation therapy is necessary for the achievement of local tumor control and impacts overall survival.

The optimal timing of chemotherapy and radiation was established by the West Japan Lung Cancer Group study (Furuse et al) and RTOG 9410 (Curran et al).[7,8] RTOG 9410 demonstrated the long-term survival benefit of the concurrent delivery of cisplatin-based chemotherapy with radiation as compared with the sequential delivery. In this three-arm randomized trial, 610 patients were randomized to either: (1) induction chemotherapy with cisplatin and vinblastine followed by 63 Gy RT in 2 Gy fractions, (2) the same chemo delivered with 63 Gy RT (2Gy/fx) concurrently, and (3) cisplatin and etoposide given concurrently with twice daily RT to 69.6 Gy (1.2 Gy/fx). Arm 2 showed the best median and overall survival (17.0 mos/16%vs 14.6 mos/10% in Arm 1, and 15.6 mos/13% in Arm 3) with similar toxicity profiles between Arms 1 and 2. In the Furuse study, 320 patients were randomized to either: (1) concurrent chemo-RT with cisplatin, vindesine, and mitomycin with RT to 56 Gy with a 10 day break after 28 Gy or (2) sequential chemo-RT with the same chemotherapy as arm 1 and RT to 56 Gy initiated after completion of chemotherapy.

This study demonstrated a 15.8% five year survival in the concurrent arm compared with a five year survival of 8.9% in the sequential chemotherapy followed by radiation therapy arm. Based on these studies, the concurrent chemo-radiation therapy is the current standard of care for the treatment of stage III unresectable NSCLC in good performance status patients; however, loco-regional recurrences and distant metastatic disease remain problematic in this patient population.

The Basis for Radiation Dose Escalation in NSCLC

One possible way to improve upon loco-regional control, which may in turn lead to decreased rates of distant metastases and improved overall survival, is radiation dose escalation. Evidence for an increased biological effect with increasing radiation doses comes from data published by Fletcher in 1973.[9] He evaluated clinical dose response curves in human epithelial tumors and based on his data and radiation oncology first principles, it is thought that doses up to 100 Gy are necessary to sterilize tumors of the size typical in NSCLC.

More recently, two studies out of the University of Michigan evaluated the relationship between biological equivalent dose (BED) and treatment outcomes in both stage I/II [10] and stage III [11] patients. Both of these studies revealed a statistically significant improvement in 5-year overall survival when the tumor received a higher BED. This relationship was independent of chemotherapy effects on overall survival in the stage III patients who received both treatments.

Clinical evidence of dose escalation leading to improved local control and survival in locally advanced NSCLC is somewhat sparse due to prior technological limitations in radiation delivery that prevented doses higher than 60-66 Gy to be delivered while meeting normal tissue toxicity constraints. RTOG 73-01 (described above) is the only published randomized trial to evaluate the dose effect on local disease control in the dose range of 40-60 Gy. Doses greater than 60 Gy were not attempted on this study because of the large radiation fields employed and the limited technology available at the time. That study did however show lower intrathoracic failure rates with higher doses of radiation.

Interestingly, survival correlated with the degree of intrathoracic tumor response to radiation. The median survival time for the patients achieving complete tumor regression was 75 weeks, in contrast to 45 weeks for those with partial regression, 36 weeks for those with stable disease, and 29 weeks for patient who progressed on therapy. Three year overall survivors after treatment was better for the patients receiving 60 Gy (approximately 15%)

compared to those treated to lower doses: 10% for 50 Gy, and 6% for 40 Gy (split or continuous).

Recently, several retrospective analyses have suggested that doses higher than 60 Gy may further improve local disease control and overall survivors. Studies from M. D. Anderson Cancer Center and Germany revealed that doses ≥ 60 Gy yield better local control rates.[12,13] Researchers from Duke and Washington Universities reported that doses ≥ 70 Gy are better.[14] In a mixed analysis of protocol and non-protocol patients, researchers from Memorial Sloan-Kettering Cancer Center reported significantly improved local control and survival with doses ≥ 64 Gy for locally advanced diseases. [15]

The 2-year local failure rates were 47% and 76% for Stage III patients treated with ≥ 64 Gy and <64 Gy, respectively. The median survival time for patients treated with ≥ 64 Gy was 20 months versus 15 months for those treated with <64 Gy.

It is important to note that the patients treated to a higher dose did not have improved outcome at the expense of greater toxicity. Both the lower dose and the higher dose groups exhibited similar esophageal and pulmonary toxicity profiles. Because of these studies, thoracic radiation oncologists have started to give a dose of 66 Gy for locally advanced lung cancer.

New Technologies that Allow for Dose Escalation

In more recent years, there have been several improvements in radiation therapy delivery that now allow for the safe delivery of higher doses to tumor while remaining within normal tissue constraints. These include computed tomography (CT)- based treatment planning and positron emission tomography (PET or PET-CT) for improved tumor delineation and conformal and intensity modulated radiation therapy for improved dose distributions. Four-dimensional (4-D) CT and image guided radiation therapy enhance knowledge of tumor motion and help limit planning target volume (PTV) margins for smaller overall radiation treatment fields. Additionally, studies have revealed that entire nodal basins did not need to be irradiated to achieve local control. Although this is not a technological advance, it has allowed for smaller clinical target volumes, which allows for dose escalation.

Dose Escalation Studies

Since the late 1990s, several phase I and II studies have explored dose escalation in the treatment of locally advanced NSCLC. RTOG 9311 employed conformal radiotherapy (CRT) to safely escalate a fractionated radiation dose to 83.8 Gy in patients who did not receive concurrent chemotherapy.[16] Several Phase I radiation dose escalation trials have been performed to test this hypothesis, primarily to determine the maximum tolerated dose in radiation therapy of NSCLC. These studies have demonstrated that 74–103 Gy (without chemotherapy) can be delivered safely if strict dose–volume limitations are applied for critical structures. [17,18,19,20,21,22]. After the establishment of safe dose escalation in stage III patients, several phase I and II trials explored the use of chemotherapy in conjunction with higher doses of RT. Hayman et al. reported that dose escalation ranging from 63 Gy to 102.9

Gy in NSCLC was safely performed using three-dimensional (3-D) CRT when the target volume was limited.[23] The median survival in Stage III NSCLC was 16 months, and the overall survival at 2 years was 36%. Socinski, et. al. increased the doses to 74 Gy using 3-D conformal radiotherapy in the treatment of Stage III NSCLC.[24] They reported that high-dose 3-D CRT of 74 Gy combined with paclitaxel and carboplatin induction chemotherapy followed by concurrent chemotherapy achieved a median survival time of 24.3 months. In a similar Phase I/II study with paclitaxel and carboplatin, Schild et al. determined that the maximum tolerated dose was 74 Gy, which achieved a median survival time of 37 months.[25] RTOG 0117 study was a phase I/II radiation dose escalation protocol in the setting of concurrent carboplatin and paclitaxel. In this study, Bradley et al reported similar results with a maximal tolerated dose of 74 Gy and median survival time of 21.6 months.[26]

Based on the results of these promising phase I/II trials, a Phase III intergroup trial (RTOG 0617/NCCTG N0628/CALGB 30609) was initiated in 2006 randomizing inoperable stage III patients to 74 Gy versus 60 Gy with concurrent carboplatin and paclitaxel given in both arms (two additional randomized arms evaluating carboplatin/paclitaxel with or without cetuximab will not be discussed here).

The dose escalation portion of the study was closed to accrual in June 2011 when a planned interim analysis showed that the higher dose arm would not provide a survival advantage over the lower dose arm with 1-yr survival rates of 70.4% and 81%, respectively. There were more deaths in the 74 Gy arm compared to the 60 Gy arm (17 versus 7), but the toxicity was equivalent between the two arms. These results were presented at the ASTRO 2011 plenary session. Further analysis is being undertaken to investigate why there was no difference in the two arms.

Future Directions

The recently presented results of RTOG 0617 beg the question, where do we go from here? One hypothesis for the lack of survival benefit in RTOG 0617 was the trial's use of what could be considered inadequate concurrent chemotherapy. Based on published data from several multi-center randomized controlled trials, platinum based chemotherapy with concurrent radiation therapy leads to improved local control and survival outcomes in patients with inoperable stage III NSCLC.

This benefit is most evident when examining the clinically significant endpoints of 3-year or 5-year overall survival rates. Cisplatin is the only drug with Phase III data available in this setting demonstrating a consistent benefit from concomitant administration with radiation. Although the concurrent application is somewhat more toxic than radiation alone, this strategy has now become feasible in the multicenter clinical practice setting where adequate supportive care measures are available and is also the recommended chemotherapy agent of choice for inoperable stage III NSCLC in the 2011 NCCN guidelines.

Most of the dose escalation trials to date, including RTOG 0617, use carboplatin-based chemotherapy based on perceived decreased toxicity compared to cisplatin, although no phase III data have supported that conclusion. It is known, however, that carboplatin is a less potent radiation sensitizer than cisplatin. Based on these data, as well as recent data from a Chinese study [27] showing improved survival with concurrent cisplatin/etoposide and radiation therapy compared to carboplatin/paclitaxel with radiation therapy, we have initiated a phase I clinical trial at our institution examining the safety of radiation dose escalation delivered concurrently with cisplatin and etoposide. We hypothesize that with improved chemotherapy, when safely delivered, will improve outcomes in inoperable stage III patients.

Conclusion

Although several prospective, randomized studies have been conducted over the last 30 years to improve the outcomes of patients with stage III inoperable NSCLC with increased use of chemotherapy, improved radiation techniques, and supportive care that allows escalation of therapy, only moderate improvements in survival have been achieved. RTOG 0617, the most recent North American trial to combine all of the elements previously shown to improve patient outcomes (concurrent chemo-RT, dose escalation), unfortunately did not show a survival benefit in the experimental 74 Gy arm. Further analysis of that trial's data is warranted to better understand why improvements in survival were not seen. Additionally, more phase I/II trials, such as the one being conducted at our institution, are necessary to identify novel treatment parameters that may improve outcomes in stage III inoperable patients.

References

[1] SEER Stat Fact Sheets: Lung and Bronchus. Surveillance Epidemiology End Results of the National Cancer Institute. Updated November 10, 2011. http://seer.cancer.gov /statfacts/html/lungb.html

[2] Roswit B, et al. The survival of patients with inoperable lung cancer: a large-scale randomized study of radiation therapy versus placebo. *Radiology*. 1968 Apr; 90(4):688-97.

[3] Pérez CA, Stanley K, Rubín P, et al. A prospective randomized study of various irradiation doses and fractionation schedules in the treatment of inoperable non oat-cell carcinoma of the lung. Preliminary report by the Radiation Therapy Oncology Group. *Cancer*. 1980; 45:2744 –2753.

[4] Perez C, Pajak T, Rubin P, et al. Long-term observations of the patterns of failure in patients with unresectable non-oat-cell carcinoma of the lung treated with definitive radiotherapy. *Cancer*. 1987; 59:1874-1881.

[5] Dillman RO, et al. A randomized trial of induction chemotherapy plus high-dose radiation versus radiation alone in stage III non-small-cell lung cancer. *N. Engl. J. Med.* 1990 Oct 4;323(14):940-5.

[6] Kubota K, Furuse K, Masaki K, et al. Role of radiotherapy in combined modality treatment of locally advanced non-small cell- lung cancer. *J. Clin. Oncol.* 1994; 12:1547–1552.

[7] Furuse K, et al. Phase III study of concurrent versus sequential thoracic radiotherapy in combination with mitomycin, vindesine, and cisplatin in unresectable stage III non-small-cell lung cancer. *J. Clin. Oncol.* 1999 Sep;17(9):2692-9.

[8] Curran WJ, et al. Sequential vs. concurrent chemoradiation for stage III non-small cell lung cancer: randomized phase III trial RTOG 9410. *J. Natl. Cancer Inst.* 2011 Oct 5;103(19):1452-60.

[9] Fletcher GH. Clinical dose response curves of human malignant epithelial tumours. *Br. J. Radiol.* 1973; 46:151.

[10] Zhao L, West BT, Hayman JA, et al. High radiation dose may reduce the negative effect of large gross tumor volume in patients with medically inoperable early-stage non-small cell lung cancer. *Int. J. Radiat. Oncol. Biol. Phys.* 2007; 68:103-10.

[11] Wang L, Correa CR, Zhao L, et al. The effect of radiation dose and chemotherapy on overall survival in 237 patients with Stage III non-small cell lung cancer. *Int. J. Radiat. Oncol. Biol. Phys.* 2009; 73:1383-90.

[12] Kupelian, PA, Komaki R, Allen P. Prognostic factors in the treatment of node-negative non–small-cell lung carcinoma with radiotherapy alone. *Int. J. Radiat. Oncol. Biol. Phys.* 996; 36:607– 613.

[13] Willner J, Baier K, Caragiani E, et al. Dose, volume, and tumor control prediction in primary radiotherapy of non–small-cell lung cancer. *Int. J. Radiat. Oncol. Biol. Phys.* 2002: 52; 382–389.

[14] Bradley JD, Ieumwananonthachai N, Purdy JA, et al. Gross tumor volume, critical prognostic factor in patients treated with three-dimensional conformal radiation therapy for non–small-cell lung carcinoma. *Int. J. Radiat. Oncol. Biol. Phys.* 2002; 52:49 –57.

[15] Rengan R, Rosenzweig KE, Venkatraman E, et al. Improved local control with higher doses of radiation in large-volume Stage III non–small-cell lung cancer. *Int. J. Radiat. Oncol. Biol. Phys.* 2004; 60:741–747.

[16] Bradley J. ea. Toxicity and outcome results of RTOG 9311: A phase I–II dose-escalation study using three-dimensional conformal radiotherapy in patients with inoperable non–small-cell lung carcinoma. *Int. J. Rad. Oncol. Biol. Phys.* 2005; 61:318-328.

[17] Robertson R.K. ea Dose escalation for non–small-cell lung cancer using conformal radiation therapy. *Int. J. Radiat. Oncol. Biol. Phys.* 1997: 37;1079–1085.

[18] Armstrong J.G. ea, Strategy for dose escalation using 3-dimensional conformal radiation therapy for lung cancer, *Ann. Oncol.* 1995: 6;693–697.

[19] Rosenzweig K.E. ea Results of a Phase I dose escalation study in the treatment of inoperable non–small-cell lung cancer. *Int. J. Radiat. Oncol. Biol. Phys.* 2003:57; S417–S418.

[20] Rosenman, J.G. ea Halle and M.A. Socinski et al., High-dose conformal radiotherapy for treatment of Stage IIIA/IIIB non–small-cell lung cancer: Technical issues and results of a Phase I/II trial. *Int. J. Radiat. Oncol. Biol. Phys.* 2002: 54; 348–356.

[21] Belderbos, J.S.A. ea Normal tissue complication probabilities for irradiation of NSCLC patients with and without elective nodal irradiation. *Lung Cancer.* 1997:18; (Suppl.) 26.

[22] Socinski M.A. ea Induction and concurrent chemotherapy with high-dose thoracic conformal radiation therapy in unresectable stage IIIA and IIIB non-small-cell lung cancer: A dose-escalation phase I trial. *J. Clin. Oncol.* 2004: 22;4341–4350.

[23] Hayman JA, Martel MK, Ten Haken RK, et al. Dose escalation in non-small-cell lung cancer using three dimensional conformal radiation therapy: Update of a phase I trial. *J. Clin. Oncol.* 2001; 19:127–136.

[24] Socinski, Mark A. et al Randomized Phase 2 Trial of Induction Chemotherapy Followed by Concurrent Chemotherapy and Dose-Escalated Thoracic Conformal Radiotherapy (74 Gy) in Stage III Non–Small-Cell Lung Cancer: CALGB 30105. *J. Clin. Oncol*. 2008: 26(15); 2457-2463.

[25] Schild S ea. Results of a phase I trial of concurrent chemotherapy and escalating doses of radiation for unresectable non-small cell lung cancer. *Int. J. Rad. Oncol. Biol. Phys*. 2005:63(2);S44.

[26] Bradley J. ea. Phase I results of RTOG 0117; a phase I/II dose intensification study using 3DCRT and concurrent chemotherapy for patients with inoperable non-small cell lung cancer. *Oncol. PASC*. 2005: 24;7063A.

[27] Hua R, Ou G, Wu S, et al. Phase II Study of Cisplatin/Etoposide vs. Weekly Paclitaxol/Carboplatin with Radiotherapy for Patients with Locally Advanced Non-small Cell Lung Cancer. *Int. J. Rad. Oncol. Biol. Phys;* 78(3), Supplement, Page S109.

In: Non-Small Cell Lung Cancer: New Research
Editor: Lina Pasquariello ISBN: 978-1-62417-804-7

Chapter 6

Mechanisms of Resistance to EGFR Inhibitors

A. López-González and M. Provencio
Hospital Universitario Puerta de Hierro-Majadahonda, Madrid, Spain

Abstract

Non small cell lung cancer (NSCLC)-specific EGFR mutations are the first target for selective treatment identified in NSCLC. The presence of EGFR mutations is a major determinant of tirosine kinase inhibitors (TKIs) response. Most of these "sensitising" mutations include exon 19 deletions, and replacement at exon 21 of leucine 858 by arginine (L858R). Despite benefits of EGFR TKIs in EGFR-mutant NSCLC, all patients develop progressive tumor growth while receiving treatment, mainly due to the development of resistance, which typically occurs after from 9 to 14 months, depending on the series [1, 2]. At least 50% of acquired TKI resistance can be attributed to a secondary mutation in the exon 20 of the EGFR gene, the T790M mutation, consisting of the substitution of a methionine residue by a threonine at position 790 of the kinase domain, which arises after exposure to TKIs [3]. Recently, intermediate and high BRCA1 baseline levels have been described as markers of shorter progression-free survival in patients treated with TKIs [4]. Other pathways that might explain acquired resistance to EGFR TKIs are the amplification of the MET oncogene [5] (which occurs independently of the T790M mutation in 20% of NSCLC) and the PI3K/Akt, MAPK [6] and NF-KB [7]. The presence of HER2 mutations is also associated with resistance to EGFR TKIs [8].

Keywords: EGFR, tyrosine kinase inhibitors, screening, resistance EGFR inhibitors

Introduction

Cancer is a major public health problem. Lung cancer is the most common cancer in the world today, both in incidence and mortality. Non-small cell lung cancer (NSCLC) accounts for approximately 80-85% of all cases of lung cancer; it has been estimated that more than 222,000 new cases will be diagnosed in the U.S. [9], and 391,000 new cases in Europe [10]. Most patients have advanced unresectable disease at the time of diagnosis and therefore have a poor prognosis. Epidemiological studies indicate little difference between prevalence and incidence, which shows the high mortality caused by this tumour [9].

Metastatic non-small-cell lung cancer is found in approximately 50% of patients at the time of diagnosis, with short survival regardless of type of chemotherapy administered. Several platinum-based chemotherapy regimens yield the similar outcomes, with median progression free survival of four months and median overall survival of 10-12 months. Due to the poor results observed after platinum-based front-line chemotherapy, research on new strategies for treatment of advanced NSCLC is warranted.

Cancer is driven by the activation and inactivation of key genes that are essential point controllers of regulatory pathways [11]. Several gene alterations are known to contribute to the development of lung cancer [12]. The recent identification of activating somatic mutations in EGFR gene, especially in lung cancer and relevance in predicting the response has resulted in increased research in this field.

Epidermal Growth Factor (EGF) was originally isolated by Cohen in 1962 [13]. In 1975 the EGF receptor (EGFR) was confirmed and in 1978 was identified as a 170 KDa protein that showed increased phosphorylation when bound to EGF in the A431 squamous cell carcinoma cell line that had an amplified EGFR gene [14]. EGFR kinase domain mutations have been identified as predictors of response to gefitinib or erlotinib.

EGFR Mutations and Clinical Implications

In 2004, three research groups identified somatic mutations in the tyrosine-kinase domain of EGFR, which were associated with high TKI-response rates [15, 16, 17]. Most of these "sensitising" mutations, which amount to about 85% of all EGFR mutations in NSCLC, include exon 19 deletions, and replacement at exon 21 of leucine 858 by arginine (L858R).

The results of numerous studies [18] have shown that these mutations were found more often in groups of patients with clinical characteristics associated with TKI sensitivity (female sex, adenocarcinomas, Asian and non-smokers).

Published data on 1,179 patients showed that over 70% of patients with EGFR mutations had TKI response, compared with 10% of patients without mutations who responded to this kind of treatment [19]. In the initial assessment by the Spanish Lung Cancer Group (SLCG), patients with mutation and second-line treatment with gefitinib had between 60-90% response, with survival close to 13 months, whereas patients without mutation had a response rate below 10% and statistically lower survival, too [20, 21].

One interesting feature is that the presence of these mutations may be associated with distinct sensitivity to TKIs. Various studies have demonstrated that both erlotinib and gefitinib are more active in patients with exon 19 deletion than in those with exon 21 mutation, with significant differences in response and survival [22, 23, 24]

The SLCG evaluated the feasibility of large-scale screening of EGFR mutations in NSCLC patients and analyzed the association between EGFR mutations and clinical outcomes to erlotinib [25].

From April 2005 through November 2008, a total of 2105 NSCLC patients from 129 institutions were prospectively screened for EGFR mutations. EGFR mutation assessment was performed centrally at the Catalan Institute of Oncology. The median time required for the EGFR mutation assay was seven days from the time the sample arrived at the laboratory until the results were reported to the investigators. Mutations in the EGFR gene were detected in 350 of 2105 patients (16.6%). Mutations were detected more frequently in women (30%), never-smokers (37.7%) and adenocarcinomas (17.3%). However, mutations were also observed in men (8.2%), former smokers (9.5%) and even in current smokers (5.8%), and in large-cell carcinomas (11.5%).

Erlotinib was administered to 217 patients, 113 of whom received erlotinib as first-line therapy and 104 as second- or third-line therapy. EGFR del 19 mutations were detected in 135 tumors, and the L858R mutation in 82 tumors. Of the 164 patients in whom EGFR mutations were also assessed in serum, 97 carried mutations: del 19 in 64 patients and L858R in 33 patients. The overall response rate was 70.6%, including 12.2% complete responses. A better response was associated with del 19 deletion mutation than with the L858R mutation (odds ratio, 3.08; 95% CI, 1.63 to 5. 81; P=0.001) and with an age between 61 and 70 years (odds ratio, 2.55; 95% CI, 1.32 to 4.96; p=0.006). Median PFS was 14 months. The duration of response was similar for patients receiving first-line or second-line therapy. Median overall survival was 27 months. Median overall survival was 28 months for patients receiving first-line therapy and 27 months for those receiving second-line therapy. Median PFS was 16 months in women and 9 months in men (P=0.003). Median overall survival was 29 months in women and 18 months in men. There were no significant differences in PFS according to performance status (PS), age, first-line versus second or third-line therapy, or smoking history.

The multivariate analysis revealed an association between poor PFS and male sex and the presence of the L858R mutation. In the multivariate analysis of overall survival, PS 1, male sex, the presence of the L858R mutation, brain metastases, and bronchioloalveolar adenocarcinoma were associated with poor prognosis.It was demonstrated that large-scale screening of patients for EGFR mutations, with subsequent customization of erlotinib is feasible and improves the outcome.

Recently two phase III trials of Asian patients with EGFR mutations, demonstrated that progression-free survival was longer for gefitinib than for those receiving chemotherapy [26, 27]. These findings show clearly that EGFR mutations are highly important in determining sensitivity to EGFR TKIs, although more prospective studies are needed to confirm their predictive and prognostic value [28].

Mechanisms of Resistance to EGFR Inhibitors

Despite benefits of EGFR TKIs in EGFR-mutant NSCLC, all patients develop progressive tumor growth while receiving treatment.

1. The T790 Mutation

The clinical efficacy of gefitinib or erlotinib is limited by the development of acquired drug resistance that is believed to be caused by the T790M mutation, which is detected in 50% of clinically resistant patients [29, 30, 31, 32].

Serial analyses of EGFR-mutated patients treated with gefitinib or erlotinib revealed the increased prevalence of the resistant T790M mutation in circulating tumor cells over time [33]. This mutation was found in about 50% of patients who suffer a relapse after initial response to EGFR TKIs, whereas its incidence is low in tumours of patients who have not received EGFR TKIs [34], but the T790M mutation has also been detected in pretreatment specimens [35]. The T790M mutation was found in pretreatment tumor samples from 10 of 26 patients (38%). The T790M mutation was associated with a strikingly short PFS – a median of 7.7 months in patients with the T790M mutation and 16.5 months in those without the mutation (hazard ratio for progression for the T790M allele, 11.5; $P<0.001$).

Irreversible EGFR inhibitors, as PF00299804, are effective in vitro and in vivo against EGFR mutant tumours that contain EGFR T790M and are currently under clinical development. Ercan D et al [36], generate models of resistance to PF00299804, using cell lines with EGFR T790M and show that the PF00299804-resistant models develop focal amplification of EGFR that preferentially involves the T790M-containing allele. They show that resistance to PF00299804 arises, at least in part, through selection of a pre-existing EGFR T790M-amplified clone both in vitro and using a xenograft model in vivo. EGFR T790M is a common resistance mechanism to both reversible, and when amplified, the irreversible EGFR kinase inhibitors further emphasizing the need to develop more potent therapies against EGFR T790M.

2. MET Pathway

MET is the receptor for hepatocyte growth factor (HGF), overexpressed in varios cancers. The amplification of the MET oncogene ocurrs independently of the T790M mutation in 20% of NSCLC.

Engelman et al [37], reported the first study of HER3 activation through a kinase other than a receptor of the EGFR family. They propose that MET amplification may promote drug resistance in other ERBB-driven cancers as well. The study describes a gefitinib-sensitive lung cancer cell line that developed resistance to gefitinib as a result of focal amplification of the MET proto-oncogene. Inhibition of MET signalling in these cells restored their sensitivity to gefitinib. MET amplification was detected in 4 of 18 (22%) lung cancer specimens that had developed resistance to gefitinib or erlotinib. They found that amplification of MET causes gefitinib resistance by driving ERBB3 (HER3)-dependent activation of PI3K, a pathway thought to be specific to EGFR/ERBB family receptors.

Turke and colleagues have suggested that EGFR TKI-resistant tumors with MET amplification arise in tumors with pre-existing clones of MET-amplified cells, which survive TKI therapy. Recently, they found the potential benefit from initial combination therapy EGFR and MET inhibition [38]. Bean [39] showed MET amplification in 21% of patients with acquired resistance to TKIs and only in 3% of untreated patients.

The overexpression of HGF, a specific ligand of MET is also involved in EGFR-TKI resistance. Yano et al administered HGF to human adenocarcinoma cell lines that harboured EGFR exon 19 deletion mutations, showing that HGF induces resistance to gefitinib in a dose-dependent manner [40]. Talking about clinical studies, it has been reported that patients with high HGF expression acquired resistance to TKIs, not having a T790M mutation or MET amplification [41]. Turke et al reported similar results when they analyzed 27 acquired resistance cases and found that HGF expression was significantly higer in the drug-resistant specimens than in the pretreatment specimens.

Recently, MET oncogene has been related with microRNAs and their role in TKI-resistant NSCLCs. MicroRNAs negatively regulate gene expression, and their dysregulation has been implicated in tumorigenesis. MiR-30b, miR-30c, miR-221 and miR-222 are modulated by both epidermal growth factor and MET receptors, and it has been shown that these miRNA have important roles in gefitinib-induced apoptosis and epithelial-mesenchymal transition of NSCLC cells in vitro and in vivo [42].

3. AKT Pathway

PI3K/Akt and MAPK represents one of most common reported causes of resistance to EGFR-targeted therapy [43]. The modulation of pAKT activity has shown to alter cellular responsiveness to chemotherapy and irradiation in NSCLC and offers opportunities for further research in clinical studies in patients with high levels of pAKT [44]. E-cadherin (epithelial marker) and vimentin are related directly and indirectly to sensitivity to TKIs [45]. Cadherins are cell surface transmembrane molecules that play a major role in epithelial cell adhesion and connect the extracellular environment to the contractile cytoskeleton leading to the activation of certain nuclear responses. In pretreating [46] resistant cell lines with the HDAC inhibitor, MS-275, induced E-cadherin along with EGFR and led to a growth-inhibitory and apoptotic effect of gefitinib similar to that in gefitinib-sensitive NSCLC cell lines including those harboring *EGFR* mutations. Thus, combined HDAC inhibitor and gefitinib treatment could represents a novel pharmacologic strategy for overcoming resistance to EGFR inhibitors in patients with lung cancer.

4. BRCA-1 Pathway

High levels of BRCA-1 (which is involved in DNA repair) has been related to wignificantly worse survival in resected non-small-cell lung cancer [47].

Relating BRCA-1 and pretreated T790M mRNA levels, Rosell et al reported a study with 129 erlotinib-treated advanced NSCLC patients with EGFR mutations [48]. The EGFR T790M mutation was observed in 35% of the patients. PFS was 12 months in patients with and 18 months in patients without the T790M mutation; PFS was 27 months in patients with low BRCA1 levels and 10 months in those with high levels. In the multivariate analysis, the presence of the T790M mutation and high BRCA1 levels were shown as markers of shorter PFS.

5. AEG-1 Pathway

Astrocyte elevated gene 1 (AEG-1) is a multifunctional oncogene which plays a role in several carcinogenic processes. AEG-1 activates IKK (which is a kinase enzyme complex part of the upstream NF-KB signal transduction cascade), leading to phosphorylation and destabilization of the NF-KB inhibitor, the gatekeeper for EGFR signalling [49].

In ASCO 2011, Viteri et al reported their study about the AEG-1 and BRCA-1 mRNA expression in 77 patients with NSCLC and EGFR mutations. They generated a risk model based in AEG-1 and BRCA-1 levels: a high risk group with patients with high levels of both genes, an intermediate-risk group with high levels of one and low levels of the other gene and a low-risk group with low levels of both genes. PFS was not reached in the low-risk group, while it was 18m for the intermediate-risk group and 8 m for the high-risk group (p=0.00006) (HR for high- vs low-risk groups, 6.6; 95%CI, 2-4-18; P<0.00001). In the multivariate analysis for PFS, the only independent prognostic variables were bone metastases (HR, 2.7; 95%CI, 1.1-6.5; P=0.03) and the AEG-1/BRCA1 risk groups (HR for high-risk group, 7.7 (95%CI, 2.8-21.3; P<0.00001) [50].

6. HER2 Pathway

The presence of HER2 mutations, described in adenocarcinoma and non-smokers [51, 52, 53] is also associated with resistance to EGFR TKIs.

In 2006 Wang et al published an article about the sensivity of TKIs in lung cancer cells with mutations in HER2/neu gene. They found that cells with a HER2 mutant were more potent that the wild type, activating signal transducers, phosphorylating EGFR and inducing survival, invasiveness and tumorigenicity, even in the presence of EGFR TKIs. Knockdown of mutant HER2 in lung cancer cells increased apoptosis and restored sensitivity to EGFR TKIs. They also found that the HER2 inhibitors lapatinib and trastuzumab inhibited growth of lung cancer cells expressing the mutant HER2 [53].

However, and also in an in vitro study, the copy number gains of HER2 has been reported related with sensitivity to gefitinib [54].

More studies are needed to clarify the role of HER2 pathway in TKIs resistance.

References

[1] Sequist LV, Martins RG, Spigel D, et al: First-line gefitinib in patients with advanced non-small-cell lung cancer harboring somatic EGFR mutations. *J Clin Oncol* 26:2442-2449, 2008

[2] Rosell R, Morán T, Carceneny E, Quiroga V et al. Non-small-cell lung cancer harbouring mutations in the EGFR kinase domain. *Clin Transl Oncol.* 2010 Feb;12(2):75-80

[3] Kobayashi S, Boggon TJ, Dayaram T, et al: EGFR mutation and resistance of non-small-cell lung cancer to gefitinib. *N Engl J Med* 352:796-792, 2005

[4] Rossell R, et al: Pretreatment EGFR T790M mutation and BRCA1 mRNA expression in erlotinib-treated advanced non-small-cell lung cancer ptients with EGFR mutations. *Clin Cancer Res.* 2011 Mar 1;17(5):1160-8.

[5] Engelman JA, Zejnullahu K, Mitsudomi T, et al. MET amplification leads to Gefitinib resistance in lung cancer by activating ERBB3 signaling. Science 2007;316:1039-1043

[6] Magne N, Fischel JL, Dubreuil A et al. Influence of epidermal growth factor receptor (EGFR), p53 and intrinsic MAP kinase pathway status of tumour cells on the antiprolifeative effect of ZD 1839 ("Iressa"). *Br J Cancer* 2006; 86: 1518-1523

[7] Bivona TG, Hieronymus H, Parker J. FAS and NF-KB signalling modulate dependence of lung cancers on mutant EGFR. *Nature.* 2011 Mar 24;471(7339):523-6.

[8] Shigematsu H, Takahashi T, Nomura M et al. Somatic mutations of the HER2 kinase domain in lung adenocarcinomas. *Cancer Res* 2005;65:1642–1646

[9] Jemal A, Siegel R, Xu J, Ward E. Cancer statistics 2010. *CA Cancer J Clin* 2010. Doi: 10.3322/caa.20073

[10] Ferlay J Parkin DM, Steliarova-Foucher E. Estimates of cancer incidence and mortality in Europe in 2008. *Eur J Cancer* 2010; 46(4): 765-81.

[11] Ding L, Getz G, Wheeler DA, et al. Somatic mutations affect key pathways in lung cancer adenocarcinoma. *Nature* 2008; 455: 1069-1075.

[12] Blanco R, Iwakawa R, Tang M, et al. A gene-alteration profile of human lung cancer cell lines. *Hum Mut.* 2009; 30:1199-206.

[13] Gschwind A, Fischer OM, Ullrich A. The discovery of receptor tyrosine kinases: targets for cancer therapy. *Nat Rev* 2004; 4: 361-370.

[14] Mitsudomi T, Ytabe Y. Epidermal growth factor receptor in relation to tumor development: EGFR gene and cancer. *FEBS Journal* 2010; 277: 301-308.

[15] Lynch TJ, Bell DW, Sordella R et al. Activating mutations in the epidermal growth factor receptor underlying response of non-small-cell lung cancer to Gefitinib. *N Engl J Med* 2004;350:2129–2139.

[16] Paez JG, Janne PA, Lee JC et al. EGFR mutations in lung cancer: Correlation with clinical response to Gefitinib therapy. *Science* 2004;304:1497–150

[17] Pao W, Miller V, Zakowski M et al. EGF receptor gene mutations are common in lung cancers from "never smokers" and are associated with sensitivity of tumors to Gefitinib and Erlotinib. *Proc Natl Acad Sci U S A* 2004; 101:13306–13311.

[18] Mitsudomi T, Kosaka T, Yatabe Y et al. Biological and clinical implications of EGFR mutations in lung cancer. *Int J Clin Oncol* 2006; 11:190-198

[19] Uramoto H, Mitsudomi T. Which biomarker predicts benefit from EGFR-TKI treatment for patients with lung cancer? *Br J Cancer* 2007; 96:857-863

[20] Cortes-Funes H, Gomez C, Rosell R, et al. Epidermal growth factor receptor activating mutations in Spanish Gefitinib-treated non-small cell lung cancer patients. *Ann Oncol* 2005;16:1081–1086

[21] Taron M, Ichinose Y, Rosell R et al. Activating mutations in the tyrosine kinase domain of the epidermal growth factor receptor are associated with improved survival in Gefitinib-treated chemorefractory lung adenocarcinomas. *Clin Cancer Res* 2005; 11:5878–5885.

[22] Mitsudomi T, Kosaka T, Endoh H et al. Mutations of the epidermal growth factor receptor gene predict prolonged survival after Gefitinib treatment in-patients with non-small-cell lung cancer with postoperative recurrence. *J Clin Oncol* 2005;23:2513–2520.

[23] Riely GJ, Pao W, Pham D et al. Clinical course of patients with non-small cell lung cancer and epidermal growth factor receptor exon 19 and exon 21 mutations treated with Gefitinib or Erlotinib. *Clin Cancer Res,* 2006; 12:839-844.

[24] Jackman DM, Yeap BY, Sequist LV et al. Exon 19 deletion mutations of epidermal growth factor receptor are associated with prolonged survival in non-small cell lung cancer patients treated with Gefitinib or Erlotinib. *Clin Cancer Res* 2006;12:3908–3914

[25] Rosell R, Morán T, Queralt C, Porta R, Cardenal F, Camps C, et al. Screening for epidermal growth factor receptor mutations in lung cancer. *N Engl J Med* 2009; 361: 958-67.

[26] Mitsudomi T, Morita S, Yatabe Y et al. Gefitinib versus cisplatin plus docetaxel in patients with non-small-cell lung cancer harbouring mutations of epidermal growth factor receptor (WJTOG 3405): an open label, randomized phase 3 trial. *Lancet Oncol* 2010; 11: 121-8

[27] Mok TS, Wu YL, Thongprasert S, Yang CH, Chu DT, et al. Gefitinib or carboplatin-paclitaxel in pulmonary adenocarcinoma. *N Engl J Med* 2009; 361: 947-957.

[28] Rosell R,Viteri S, Molina MA, Benlloch S, Tarón M. Epidermal growth factor receptor tyrosine kinase inhibitors as first-line treatment in advanced nonsmall-cell lung cancer. *Curr Opin Oncol* 2010; 22: 112-120.

[29] Pao W, Miller VA, Politi KA et al. Acquired resistance of lung adenocarcinomas to Gefitinib or Erlotinib is associated with a second mutation in the EGFR kinase domain. *PLoS Med* 2005;2:1–11.

[30] Kobayashi S, Boggon TJ, Dayaram T et al. EGFR mutation and resistance of non-small-cell lung cancer to Gefitinib. *N Engl J Med* 2005;352:786–792.

[31] Nguyen KS, Kobayashi S, Costa DB. Acquired resistance to epidermal growth factor receptor tyrosine kinase inhibitors in non-small-cell lung cancers dependent on the epidermal growth factor receptor pathway. *Clin Lung Cancer* 2009; 10: 281-289.

[32] Zhou W, Ercan D, Chen L, Yun CH, Li D, et al. Novel mutant-selective EGFR kinase inhibitors against EGFR T790M. *Nature* 2009; 462: 1070-1074.

[33] Maheswaran S, Sequist LV, Nagrath S, Ulkus L, Brannigan B, et al. Detection of mutations in EGFR in circulating lung-cancer cells. *N Engl J Med* 2008; 359: 366-377.

[34] Toyooka S, Kiura K, Mitsudomi T. EGFR mutation and response of lung cancer to Gefitinib. *N Engl J Med* 2005; 352:2136.

[35] Inukai M, Toyooka S, Ito S, Asano H, Ichihara S, et al. Presence of epidermal growth factor receptor gene T790M mutation as a minor clone in non-small cell lung cancer. *Cancer Res* 2006; 66: 7854-7858.

[36] Ercan D, Zejnullahu K, Yonesaka K, et al. Amplification of EGFR T790M causes resistance to an irreversible EGFR inhibitor. *Oncogen*e 2010 feb 1. Epub a head.

[37] Engelman JA, Zejnullahu K, Mitsudomi T, et al. MET amplification leads to Gefitinib resistance in lung cancer by activating ERBB3 signaling. *Science* 2007;316:1039-1043

[38] TurkeAB, ZejnullahuK, Wu YL, et al. Preexistence and clonal selection of MET amplification in EGFR mutant NSCLC. *Cancer Cell* 2010; 19: 77-88.

[39] Bean J, Brennan C, Shih JY et al. MET amplification occurs with or without T790M mutations in EGFR mutant lung tumors with acquired resistance to Gefitinib or Erlotinib. *PNAS* 2007; 104:20932-20937

[40] Yano S, Wang W, Li QI, et al. Hepatocyte growth factor induces gefitinib resistance of lung adenocarcinoma with epidermal growth factor receptor-activating mutations. *Cancer Research.* 2008;68(22):9479–9487

[41] Kosaka T, Yamaki E, Mogi A et al. Mechanisms of resistance to EGFR TKIs and development of a new generation of drugs in non-small-cell lung cancer. *J Biomed Biotechnol.* 2011;2011:165214. Epub 2011 Jun 2

[42] Garofalo M, Romano G, Di Leva G, et al. EGFR and MET receptor tyrosine kinase-altered microRNA expression induces tumorigenesis and gefitinib resistance in lung cancers. Nat Med. 2011; Dec 11. doi:20-1038/nm.Magne N, Fischel JL, Dubreuil A et al. Influence of epidermal growth factor receptor (EGFR), p53 and intrinsic MAP kinase pathway status of tumour cells on the antiprolifeative effect of ZD 1839 ("Iressa"). *Br J Cancer* 2006; 86: 1518-1523.

[44] Schuurbiers OCJ, Kaanders JHAM, van der Heijden HFM, et al. The PI3K/AKT-pathway and radiation resistance mechanisms in Non-small cell lung cancer. *J Thorac Oncol* 2009; 4: 761-767.

[45] Thomson S, Buck E, Petti F, et al. Epithelial to mesenchymal transition is a determinant of sensitivity of non-small-cell lung carcinoma cell lines and xenografts to epidermal growth factor receptor inhibition. *Cancer Res* 2005; 65:9455-9462

[46] Witta SE, Gemmill RM, Hirsch FR, et al. Restoring e-cadherin expression increases sensitivity to epidermal growth factor receptor inhibitors in lung cancer cell lines. *Cancer Res* 2006; 66:944-950

[47] Rosell R et al. BRCA1: a novel prognostic factor in resected non-small-cell lung cancer. *Plos One.* 2007; 2(11): e1129

[48] Rosell R et al, Pretreatment EGFR T790M mutation and BRCA1 mRNA expression in erlotinib-treated advanced non-small-cell lung cancer patients with EGFR mutations. *Clin Cancer Res.* 2011 Mar 1;17(5):1160-8.

[49] Häcker H, Karin M (October 2006). "Regulation and function of IKK and IKK-related kinases". *Sci. STKE* 2006 (357): re13.

[50] Viteri S et al. Astrocyte elevated gene 1 (AEG-1) mRNA expression in non-small cell lung cancer patients with epidermal growth factor receptor (EGFR) mutations. 2011 ASCO Annual Meeting Abstract No:105421

[51] Shigematsu H, Takahashi T, Nomura M et al. Somatic mutations of the HER2 kinase domain in lung adenocarcinomas. *Cancer Res* 2005;65:1642–1646.

[52] Stephens P, Hunter C, Bignell G et al. Lung cancer: Intragenic ERBB2 kinase mutations in tumours. *Nature* 2004;431:525–526.

[53] Han SW, Kim TY, Jeon YK et al. Optimization of patient selection for Gefitinib in non-small cell lung cancer by combined analysis of epidermal growth factor receptor mutation, K-ras mutation, and Akt phosphorylation. *Clin Cancer Res* 2006;15:12:2538–2544.

[54] Wang SE, Narasanna A, Pérez-Torres M et al. Her2 kinase domain mutation results in constitutive phosphorylation and activation of HER2 and EGFR and resistance to EGFR tyrosine kinase inhibitors. *Cancer Cell.* 2006 Jul:10(1):25-38

[55] Gandhi J, Zhang J, Xie Yet al. Alterations in genes of the EGFR signaling pathway and their relationship to EGFR tyrosine kinase inhibitor sensitivity in lung cancer cell lines. *PLoS One.* 2009;4(2):e4576. Epub 2009 Feb 24.

Index

A

B

C

D

H

I

J

K

L

M

N

O

P

Q

R

S

T

U

V

W

X

Y

Z